WHY DON' YOU H

GU00394382

HARLEY STREET SPECIALIST TELLS ALL

WHAT DOCTORS, DRUG COMPANIES AND POLITICIANS DON'T WANT YOU TO KNOW!

THE SIMPLE 'DRUG FREE' WAY TO GOOD HEALTH

GERARD KIELTY I.R.B; I.D.E.

OVER 50 DIFFERENT HEALTH PROBLEMS CURED IN WEEKS WITHOUT DRUGS!

WHY DOCTORS DON'T MAKE YOU HEALTHY.

Published by:
Chipmukapublishing ltd
PO Box 6872
Brentwood
Essex
CM13 1ZT
United Kingdom

www.chipmunkapublishing.com

Copyright © 2006 Gerard Kielty

ISBN 978 1 84747 000 3

Printed on recycled paper
Every tree saved is vital to our planet and its people

THIS BOOK IS BASED ON THE *TRUE-LIFE* EXPERIENCE OF AUTHOR MR GERARD KIELTY I.R.B; I.D.E.

THIS BOOK EXPLAINS HOW WITH A SIMPLE CHANGE OF DIET 80% OR MORE OF OUR EVERYDAY HEALTH PROBLEMS ARE EASILY CURED *WITHOUT* DOCTORS OR DRUGS OF ANY KIND.

ALL REFERENCE TO HEALTH AND FOOD INTOLERANCE IS BASED ON FACT.

THIS STORY ALSO SHOWS THE HIGH LEVEL OF RESISTANCE THAT EXISTS IN BOTH MEDICAL AND POLITICAL CIRCLES TO ANY FORM OF HEALTHCARE THAT ACTUALLY WORKS.

A GREAT BARRIER KNOWN AS *THE ESTABLISHMENT* HAS BEEN CREATED OVER MANY GENERATIONS.

IT PROTECTS *'INCOMPETENT'* DOCTORS FROM FEAR OF PROSECUTION AND ALLOWS DRUG COMPANIES TO CONTINUE TO IGNORE ADVANCED AND PROVEN HEALTHCARE TECHNOLOGY.

SUCH TECHNOLOGY WOULD APPEAR TO BE SEEN AS A MAJOR THREAT TO THEIR HUGE PROFITS.

PROFITS THAT RUN INTO BILLIONS EVERY YEAR FROM THE PRESCRIBING OF UNNECESSARY DRUGS.

THIS BOOK LOOKS IN DETAIL AT DOCTORS THAT KILL HUNDREDS OF PATIENTS EVERY DAY THROUGH GROSS INCOMPETENCE.

MOST DOCTORS.... I HOPE AND BELIEVE HAVE OUR BEST INTERESTS AT HEART.
IT JUST WORRIES ME TO THINK THAT IF DRUG COMPANIES MADE PEOPLE HEALTHY THEY WOULD GO OUT OF BUSINESS.

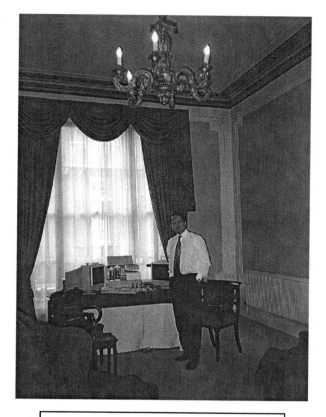

Figure 1: Mr Kielty at his Harley Street Clinic

Mr Kielty is qualified to American Food and Drugs Administration standards and is a leading specialist in the field of Electro-Dermal Screening. His credentials have been signed by the US Secretary of State Madeleine K. Albright.

WHY DOCTORS DON'T MAKE YOU HEALTHY.

WHY DOCTORS DON'T MAKE YOU HEALTHY.

****

This book is dedicated to a very special lady called Wilma. Thanks for all your help since the birth of Health Scan. Thanks for your endless support over the years and thanks for helping thousands of people to become healthy through the work that we do.

6 Dec 2007.

To Vicky,

I wish you a lifetime of good health.

Regards.

Gerard

WHY DOCTORS DON'T MAKE YOU HEALTHY.

Foreword by practising GP
Dr. Desmond Spence

Founder of the NO FREE LUNCH organisation and tutor of medicine at Glasgow University

Only a few years ago like most doctors I was up to my neck in hospitality and freebies. One night, however, I returned from speaking at a meeting clutching a large cheque from a pharmaceutical company and feeling rather self-important. My Glaswegian born wife, who does not suffer fools gladly was disgusted and told me that she preferred the snivelling medical student she met 15 years before in a pub, pulling pints for £1.80 an hour, to the corporate pawn I had become. She pointed out that they were paying for my influence, not my wit or charisma.

On reflection, I couldn't deny it. Why hadn't I seen it before? As a student I took countless freebies and thought the industry was fantastic. As a junior doctor I went with my colleagues to some of the most exclusive restaurants in Glasgow and got drunk at the drug companies expense.
In general practice they provided my lunch on a daily basis. Company representatives sponsored my practice meetings and even paid for, and attended our Christmas parties. I also conducted research for which I was paid a great deal of money. All these things influenced which drugs I prescribed to my patients. I felt beholden to the drug representatives and would always prescribe their more expensive medications. In my defence, I can merely say that I was only doing what everybody else did. One of the most frightening strangleholds the pharmaceutical companies have on the

medical profession is the invaluable resources it provides for research.

This can involve tens of millions of pounds being paid to hospitals that become dependant on this money. The drug companies own the research and control the interpretation of results. A spin is put on positive findings while negative news is suppressed. This research is published in leading medical journals which, in turn, depend on drug companies to survive. Both the British Medical Journal and The Lancet receive huge sums from the drug industry in advertising revenue. When 'research' is published, top NHS doctors and influential journalists are often flown to five star hotels for international drug launches.

These all-expenses-paid trips are passed off as *'educational.'* Drug companies allocate £10,000 a year for marketing their products to each GP in the UK.

Doctors rely heavily on information supplied by the pharmaceutical industry. But proper research suggests that just six per cent of this information is supported by hard evidence. All this leads to another important issue - we the public are taking record levels of drugs but our health is not improving. I see some patients who take more than ten medications a day and I feel that these multiple drugs may do a lot more harm than good. The pharmaceutical industry has invested a fortune in making us sick and neurotic.

Put bluntly, the profit motive of the pharmaceutical industry is corrupting doctors and destroying society's sense of well being. The medical profession continues to be in denial over the influence of the pharmaceutical industry. Many doctors are addicted to its hospitality and freebie culture, so beware; your prescription may not have been issued for all the right reasons.

<u>HEALTH PROBLEMS CURED</u>

IF YOU SUFFER FROM ANY OF THE FOLLOWING AILMENTS THEN THIS BOOK IS FOR YOU.

**Arthritis - Asthma - Athletes Foot
Bloated Stomach
Blood Pressure problems
Catarrh - Colitis - Concentration
Constipation - Coughing - Cramp
Crohn's Disease
Chronic Fatigue Syndrome (M.E)
Depression - Dermatitis - Diarrhoea
Dizziness
Eczema - Epilepsy - Eye Sensitivity
Gout - Tourette Syndrome
Haemorrhoids - Hay fever - Headaches
Heartburn
Hot Flushes - Hyperactivity
Irritability - Irritable Bowel Syndrome
Lack of Libido - Leg Ulcers
Lethargy - Loss of Sense of Smell
Loss of Confidence
Memory Loss - Migraine - Mood Swings
Sleep problems**

cont

**Mouth Ulcers - Nausea
Palpitations - Panic Attacks
Pre-menstrual Tension
Rhinitis - Sciatica
Sinusitis - Sneezing
Snoring - Stress - Sweating
Thrush - Tinnitus
Vomiting - Weight Gain or Loss**

Testimonial letters on file and quoted throughout this book prove that a **'SINGLE'** Health Scan food intolerance test **(NOT AN ALLERGY TEST)** has cured the above health problems. These results have been achieved continuously throughout the scanning of approximately 10,000 patients.

All references in this book regarding health or individuals is based on fact and can be supported by documentary evidence. Client names have been changed to protect their identity.

QUOTATIONS FROM A FEW OF OUR TESTIMONIAL LETTERS

"Thank you for giving me back my life!"

"I find it amazing that after years of suffering that there is absolutely nothing wrong with me anymore and it was all so simple. I don't think I have ever felt so healthy I just wish I did this years ago."

"I thank god for the day I went to Health Scan."
(CATHOLIC PRIEST)

"Its amazing just how well your brain can and will run your body!… When you **'stop'** poisoning it!"

"After such nagging pain for so long I can hardly believe that it has gone, nevertheless its true! A thousand thanks for helping me to overcome my debilitating complaint."

"Within about 5 days I noticed a dramatic improvement and within 2 weeks the symptoms had almost disappeared completely."

"I feel a vitality I thought I'd lost forever years ago. It's like waking up and coming out of a fog."

"As you can see the information from the scan has proved both accurate and useful, and I have strongly recommended your scan to other headache sufferers."

"Before my scan I had constant IBS, headaches and skin problems. I feel that I can now truthfully say that it is the best money I have ever spent."

"I have not had to use my inhaler once. I am so delighted that my Asthma is now a thing of the past. I cannot recommend Health Scan enough."

"I was crippled with pain and cannot believe that it has gone."

"Cured in one pain free hour, your work is amazing you really are a sanity saver."

"I think having the Health Scan was a turning point in my life. It was and will be the best thing I ever did."

Contents

Page

PART 4: WHY DOCTORS DON'T MAKE YOU HEALTHY!

Figures

WHY DOCTORS DON'T MAKE YOU HEALTHY.

HEALTH SCAN

THE FUTURE OF MEDICINE

THIS BOOK WILL CURE MILLIONS OF PEOPLE AND CHANGE THE WORLD OF HEALTHCARE FOR EVER

PART ONE

THE LEGAL DRUG BARONS

This book is written without prejudice

WHY DOCTORS DON'T MAKE YOU HEALTHY.

Chapter 1

INTRODUCTION

This might be a good time to tell you a little about myself and how I came to be in this business. I originally worked in radiography, I had planned to become a doctor but working with medical students put me off that idea.

Why?

Well, I guess that I saw a lot of what went on in the background and I didn't like it.

What do I mean?

I just felt that students were being brainwashed, they were taught a certain way of working and if they questioned it they were either pushed back into line or out the door. Most of the time they were not allowed to think for themselves and if they rocked the boat they were certainly out. So basically by the time they had struggled through Medical School they had learnt to go along with the status quo and the drug companies; any inclination they might have had previously to rebel had long since been knocked out of them. So these young doctors came out into the big wide world of medicine as shining examples of our National Health Service training and went on to write *thousands* of questionable prescriptions for the rest of their days. Not necessarily making their patients better but definitely making the drug companies richer. I didn't know about food intolerance in those days but I instinctively knew that medication was *not* always the answer, as the corridors of my hospital were full of patients that were on medication. All medical students are trained by doctors and learn from books (mostly) written by doctors. So these young students all graduate from medical school with more or less the same indoctrination and beliefs. Good and bad practices were/are passed on from generation to generation and students have to accept them if they are to pass exams and eventually practice medicine. Once they have become part of the **'Establishment'** it is extremely difficult for them to break away from the accepted policy, especially if they wish to progress in their career. The low pay and long hours leave little time for introspection and even if there was still a lingering desire to try and change the system it is unlikely that they would have the time or energy.

I didn't like what I saw going on around me so I decided to follow a different career. After radiography I worked for a time in cardiology before becoming a paramedic. I enjoyed paramedic work very much, believe it or not I still miss the thrill of working at the sharp end and having to make instant decisions that make the difference between life and death, but what I don't miss is the low pay.

One day about ten years ago I made up my mind that I would try and make a more lucrative living and the only way I could do that was to work for myself. I had been working with the human body throughout my career and I probably knew it better than most doctors. So I decided to take this knowledge a stage further and studied nutrition and the effects of food and allergens on the body. I set up my own clinic but after a while I felt that the general advice available to patients was a bit of a lottery (just as it is when a doctor writes a prescription) because if you think about it health advice, medication and nutritional advice is a bit of a numbers game. What I mean is if a doctor gives the same advice and or medication to 100 people who are suffering from the same health problem, some would get better, some would get worse and some would stay the same. Even with all their training and their wealth of medical knowledge the doctor still has to make an **'educated'** guess when it comes to diagnosis and medication. The fact is that every patient is an individual and they will all react in different ways to the same medication, advice or even food. With the system that exists at the moment the best a patient can hope for is a pill to give them some relief, it's very rare that they are cured and more often than not the patient will end up with some very unpleasant side effects. I always felt that there had to be a solution other than pills (which only mask the symptoms) and at long last I found that solution in the amazing world of food intolerance. The difference between treating every patient with a tailor made health plan as opposed to the same old medication is remarkable. Every Health Scan patient in the last ten years had already been to see their doctor and in many cases several hospital **'specialists'** also, many had waited months for an appointment and even then they didn't get to see the specialist but were fobbed off with his or her underling after hours of sitting in a draughty hospital corridor with dozens of other poor hopefuls. On top of that they were mostly treated as inferior and not encouraged to waste the doctor's **'valuable time'** by asking too many questions.

One of the arguments that are used by the medical profession is that they simply cannot handle their enormous workload and that they need the government to pour in more money and resources. The problem that I have with this argument is that most of the health problems that the medical profession is overloaded with can be treated simply and without drugs as I have proved about 10,000 times. If this technology were used by the NHS it would allow doctors to concentrate on those patients with critical life threatening conditions and it would cure literally millions of people suffering from nothing more than a dietary related problem in the form of food intolerance. My work with more than 10,000 patients has proved beyond doubt that doctors and drugs are **not** required to treat most everyday health problems.

WHY DOCTORS DON'T MAKE YOU HEALTHY.

A doctor's time could be put to better use looking after the serious end of healthcare and the taxpayers money currently wasted on unnecessary drugs could definitely be better invested.

Chapter **2**

WHAT IS FOOD INTOLERANCE?

Let me explain it to you.

Have you ever seen a healthy looking drug addict?

No!

Well!...**'food'** is a drug!... and as such it poisons the brain just like any conventional drug would!
Heroin grows in the ground!...So does a lettuce!
So why is a lettuce not a drug also?

It is!

Here is my definition of a drug:

Anything that enters the body through skin absorption or by being inhaled, injected, eaten or drunk.

Everything that enters the body **will** have a positive or negative effect **on** the brain. Some of these **drugs** will cause the brain to malfunction and others will be acceptable. Every brain will work better if you do not give it drugs that cause it to malfunction. When a brain is allowed to work properly in this way it then runs the body properly and most health problems clear up without the need for medication of any sort.

As mentioned in my definition above you can **inhale** drugs or **absorb** them through your skin! You can **inject** drugs and of course you can also **eat** and **drink** them. Well, when people eat or drink certain drugs or **foods** if you prefer to call them that their brain will often become intolerant to them or to be more specific their brain will have a problem with the **electrical signal** that is given off by the food. We often hear people saying they are comfort eating, in other words they feel better when they've eaten certain foods.

Well drug addicts feel better when they've had a fix!
There's **no** difference! Heroin sends a signal to your brain and so does chicken. The only thing is that they each send a **different** signal for the very simply reason that heroin and chicken are different chemicals once they break down in your body. If you got up every day of your life and **deliberately** poisoned your brain you wouldn't expect to be healthy.

Would you?

Well you're doing that **and** so is everyone else out there in this big wide world.
Let me explain. We need electricity in our body but we don't generate it, so therefore we have to put it in and we do through the foods we eat each and every day. All foods that enter our body break down and become chemicals. These chemicals then release a **unique** electrical signal which gets picked up in our **nervous system** and goes straight to our brain.
If we don't eat. We die! What actually happens is that we run **out** of electricity. We run **flat** just as any battery would.
Without electricity in our body our brain **and** heart stop, we're then waiting for paramedics to rush in and defibrillate us. They **jump start** us like a car with a flat battery, that's the first thing they do. They put electricity **into** our body, the electricity passes around our nervous system in a split second and shocks our brain into action. In that same split second our brain sends out a signal

to kick-start the heart. There's no way that they could start up our **heart** if they didn't start up our **brain** first because our brain sends out the signal to make our heart work. Our **brain** sends out the signals to make **everything** in our body work.

The reason that defibrillation is performed above the heart is because it's a flattish surface and a great place to get a good connection with the nervous system.

You can't expect to get a good connection on the head because it's round and normally there's hair in the way. Basically, it would make no difference **where** you connect to put electricity into the body it would still pass through the nervous system and start the brain first.

So to recap, what I'm saying here is that we need electricity in our body but we don't generate it, we actually get it from food.

Take a look at the potato clock on the next page as it proves my point perfectly. You can buy these in any high street in the UK. There are no batteries in this clock it runs off the **electricity** that comes from the potatoes. But it will run off **any** food you wish to plug it into and that's where we get the electricity from that keeps us alive, if we don't eat **we die**. What actually happens is that we run out of electricity over a few months or so and our **brain** shuts down.

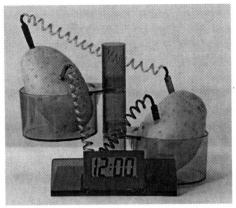

Potato powered clock

Figure 2
Potato Powered Clock

I do have to change the potatoes every two or three-week's though because they lose their charge, just like any battery would. A potato or anything else is only a carrier of an **electrical signal** as far as our nervous system is concerned. As I said before it doesn't matter if it's a potato, a piece of chicken, a pill from the doctor or heroin they all break down in our body become chemicals and send out a **unique** electrical signal.

This signal then gets picked up in our nervous system and goes straight to our brain. That's **all** that arrives at our brain, **nothing else** just the **electrical signal** from that item.
The clever part though is that they all send out **different** electrical signals. An apple will send out a **different** signal than an orange for the very simple reason that they're **different** chemicals. So as I've just said, if we didn't put food into our body we would run

flat like a battery and die within a few months, because it's the electricity **from** the food that actually keeps us alive.

At this point you could be forgiven for thinking that I am talking about food allergies....well I'm not!

There is **no** comparison between a food allergy and a food intolerance. An allergy occurs in the **'Immune System'**.... whereas an intolerance occurs in the **'Nervous System'** and these are two completely **different** systems in your body.

An allergy condition is brought about when two or more chemicals (foods etc) meet in your body and react in a negative way. This can also happen when your glands squirt out chemistry if you get a foreign invader in your bloodstream, it's your bodies **natural defence mechanism** coming into play. If you get a protein for example: an undigested food particle or a bug in your bloodstream then your glands will kick out chemicals and try to kill these off before they get to your vital organs and cause serious damage or even death.

A foreign body which activates an allergic response is known as an antigen. If your immune system cannot fight the invader then you would normally be given a course of antibiotics.

Allergies occur in your **immune system** whereas an intolerance occurs in your **nervous system**.... in other words in your **brain**. But remember it's your brain that **controls** your immune system so if your brain is not working properly then how can your immune system. Food intolerance is the **electrical resistance** in your brain to a specific signal that is given off by a food or any other item that enters your body.

Food intolerance occurs when your **brain** gets fed up with certain signals from certain foods and it simply can't handle them anymore. This can happen when you're 1 or 91…there are no rules, we're all individuals and we all have our own **unique** brain.

As a result of putting **wrong** signals into your brain (that computer in your head) it then sends out **wrong** signals just as any computer would. These wrong signals then run down wires called nerves that lead **anywhere** they wish to in your body and that's what causes **80%** of everyday health problems.

Your brain **is** a computer! It's the best computer on the planet.
It controls almost everything that happens in your body and just like any computer if you give it problems, then it gives you problems.

I've scanned thousands of people and I have yet to find a person that does not have some intolerance to some of the foods that they are eating on a daily basis. Although we know that an allergy can kill, in my experience not many people have allergies that cause much in the way of health problems. What they **all** have though is an intolerance to **some** of their regular daily foods and that's where **most** of their health problems are coming from. Probably 35-40% of the people I've treated over the years had already been to their local hospital for an allergy test. It obviously didn't work or they wouldn't have needed me. The reason it didn't work is that the doctors were looking in the wrong place for the answers, they were checking the **Immune System** for allergic response when they should have been checking the **Nervous System** for electrical resistance, in other words for **Food Intolerance**.

Remember!

An allergy occurs in the **'Immune system'**... whereas an intolerance occurs in the **'Nervous system'**....and these two systems are totally different.

Chapter **3**

THE TEST

It is possible to be allergic to certain foods and not to be intolerant to them. (and visa-versa) We all know how a doctor tests for allergies but let me now explain how a food intolerance test is carried out.

The testing is drug free, pain free and non-invasive, as no medical examination is required. My computer has over 40,000 signals programmed into it. These are signals from foods, chemicals animals, dusts etc. These signals are sent out one at a time to your brain by me pressing a probe gently **onto** an acupuncture point on your finger. This point is a direct electrical link to your brain so in this way we get the most accurate feedback.

In so doing I'm measuring your brains resistance to a specific signal with the worlds most advanced ohmmeter which is built into my computer.

For example if I wished to test your intolerance to chicken I would call up the signal for chicken and the word would appear on my screen. I would then touch your finger with the probe from my computer and send the same signal to your brain that it would receive if you were to eat chicken. We then get an instant numerical **resistance** reading back from your brain. In this way we know immediately to what extent your brain **can** or **cannot** handle the signal from chicken.

If it shows a reading between 48 and 57 on my screen then there is no major resistance and you can eat chicken. The nearer it is to 50 the better the signal/food suits your brain.

If it shows a reading 47 or less or 58 or more then your brain **cannot** handle the signal from chicken...so don't eat it.

(There are some sample printouts on the following pages)

Remember!...It's your **brain** that runs your body...not your taste buds or your stomach...So it makes sense to keep your **brain** happy.

Your brain talks to you every second of every day, if you give it problems then it will give you problems...It's as simple as that.

WHY DOCTORS DON'T MAKE YOU HEALTHY.

```
Item Readings Report :  A.SAMPLE
Wed Jul 26 13:17:11 2006   Tested by G KIELTY
```

	Item Name	ID	Max	
1.	Wheat, bran	001	81	
2.	Wheat, whole	002	77	
3.	Cod	003	75	**ITEMS CURRENTLY**
4.	Carrot	004	74	**NOT ACCEPTABLE**
5.	Banana	005	68	**TO YOUR SYSTEM**
6.	Asparagus	006	64	
7.	Butter	007	63	
8.	Lactose	008	62	
9.	Pepper, black	009	62	
10.	Pear	010	57	
11.	Coffee	011	57	
12.	Tea	012	56	
13.	Sugar	013	56	
14.	Milk, cows	014	56	
15.	Oil, Sunflower	021	55	
16.	Rye	022	55	
17.	Egg, White	024	55	
18.	Apple	026	55	
19.	Curry	027	55	
20.	Garlic	029	55	
21.	Oil, olive	031	55	
22.	Orange	033	54	
23.	Margarine	035	54	
24.	Rice	036	54	**ITEMS CURRENTLY**
25.	Milk, goats	037	54	**ACCEPTABLE**
26.	Milk, soya	038	54	**TO YOUR SYSTEM**
27.	Grape	039	54	
28.	Beef	042	54	
29.	Wine, white	043	54	
30.	Chicken	044	54	
31.	Grapefruit	045	54	
32.	Olive	046	53	
33.	Salt	047	53	
34.	Yoghurt, cow	048	52	
35.	Chocolate	049	52	
36.	Crab	050	52	
37.	Oat	051	51	
38.	Cheese, cheddar	054	51	
39.	Tuna	056	51	
40.	Egg, Whole	857	51	
41.	Cheese, cottage	058	51	
42.	Strawberry	062	51	
43.	Bean, Haricot (Navy/Pinto)	063	51	
44.	Lamb/mutton	064	51	
45.	Pork	065	51	
46.	Chilli	066	51	
47.	Bean, Kidney	067	51	
48.	Lentil, red	068	51	
49.	Ham	069	50	
50.	Bean, Soya	070	50	
51.	Broccoli	078	50	
52.	Yeast, bakers	079	50	
53.	Egg, Yolk	081	49	
54.	Yeast, brewers	082	49	
55.	Almond	083	49	
56.	Wine, red	086	49	
57.	Corn	089	48	

Figure 3A: Sample Printout of a Health Scan Food Test Report.
(Top Half of Report).

```
Item Readings Report :  A.SAMPLE
Wed Jul 26 13:35:36 2006   Tested by G KIELTY
```

	Item Name	ID	Max	
1.	BASIL	HBO8	75	**ITEMS CURRENTLY**
2.	GINSENG	HBO9	75	**NOT ACCEPTABLE**
3.	CHAMOMILE	HB23	73	**TO YOUR SYSTEM**
4.	FENNEL	HB25	56	
5.	NICOTINE	HB26	56	
6.	LAVENDER	HB30	55	
7.	SAFFRON	HB31	54	
8.	ROSEMARY	HB34	54	
9.	TARRAGON	HB39	53	
10.	THYME	HB38	53	
11.	TURMERIC	HB44	53	
12.	DOG HAIR	HB57	53	
13.	BAY	HB66	53	
14.	CINNAMON	HB68	53	
15.	CLOVE	HB77	53	**ITEMS CURRENTLY**
16.	CAT HAIR	HB78	51	**ACCEPTABLE**
17.	KLEENEX	HB79	51	**TO YOUR SYSTEM**
18.	CAT EPITHELIUM	HB87	51	
19.	FEATHER, GOOSE	HB89	50	
20.	PARSLEY	HB90	50	
21.	DILL	AD02	50	
22.	OREGANO	AD02a	50	
23.	FEATHER, DUCK	AD05	50	
24.	MARJORAM	AD05a	50	
25.	LANOLINE	AD07	49	
26.	FEATHER, MIX	AD09	49	
27.	DOG EPITHELIUM	AD10	49	
28.	GINGER	QM022	48	
29.	COMFREY	CO07	48	
30.	SAGE	AF158	45	
31.	CORIANDER (CILANTRO)	AF071	40	
32.	CRANBERRY	V314	34	**ITEMS CURRENTLY**
33.	COD LIVER OIL	HS309	31	**NOT ACCEPTABLE**
34.	PEPPERMINT	EP27	23	**TO YOUR SYSTEM**
35.	SPEARMINT	HB57	21	
36.	EUCALYPTUS	HS208	20	

Figure 3B: Sample Printout of other Items
Regularly Tested at Health Scan

In a normal food intolerance test I scan for about 180 everyday foods. It takes about an hour to run through them and we end up with an instant printout that's been written by **your** brain, it doesn't get more accurate than that. And quite frankly if you do not listen to your own brain then **who's** brain are you going to listen to?

There's no human being on this planet that can tell you what foods suit their **own** brain when it comes to food intolerance so how are they going to advise you about yours? Talking to humans is a complete waste of time.

Remember: Your brain is unique!...Just like your fingerprint.

It's simple really...when you don't eat the **wrong** foods your brain starts sending out the **right** signals and within a month or so all sorts of health problems clear up...and if you don't have a problem then you don't need medication. So you can see why drug companies don't like this technology one little bit.

Drug companies are probably the biggest companies in the world and they didn't get there by making people healthy. Think about it...drug companies make **nothing** out of healthy people so from a business point of view why would they want to cure you? I'm not saying here that drug companies deliberately don't cure people otherwise they would sue me but it is an interesting thought don't you agree?

A single food intolerance test clears **all** your health problems in one go because for the first time in your life (with respect) your brain is working properly as it's not being poisoned. So it sends out the right signals for once. Children generally recover quicker than adults, I guess it's because they have had less time to create the problem in the first place.

A question I'm often asked is: Can I test a food even if the patient has never eaten it?

Yes!…The scan will test the effect on your brain from **any** item even if you have never put it into your body.

Age has got nothing to do with feeling good, people around 50 or 60 generally accept that they are getting old and act accordingly. Around this time of life most people get lots of aches and pains and think that it's just their body getting past it. Well that's not the case. It's just that you've been poisoning your brain with bad drugs for 50 or 60 years and your brain has had enough.

So it tells you!

If you stop poisoning your brain every day then it will wake up and not only will your general health problems disappear but your energy and concentration levels will go through the roof. You will feel 20 years younger within a few months. When we were kids we thought that anybody over 40 or so was old. But as oldies know they are still kids at heart, it's just that the years go by and we can't stop time. Inside every **older body** there's a young person trapped. Well! When you follow your scan then you feel **great** every minute of the day and that young person returns once more. There's nothing worse than pain or just feeling generally unhealthy to make a person miserable and to make the people closest to you miserable also.

Most people have a scan once a year to keep in peak condition. It's no different than taking your car to the garage for a tune up. You don't service your car **once** and then expect it to run perfectly for the next 50 or 60 years…well it's the same with your brain. Things **will** change, we are walking chemistry sets. If they didn't change then you wouldn't get healthy in the first place. But if you keep an annual eye on the situation you can continue to stay healthy.

38

Does the probe hurt?

No!... I scan four year olds and they love every minute of it.
I don't **puncture** the skin I just press the probe gently **onto** the skin and that connects me to your brain, you feel nothing else. The scanning system I use was developed by doctors and computer experts. It was invented in America some twenty years ago and it underwent eight years of clinical trials before being granted a licence by the American Food and Drugs Administration. The FDA are the toughest licensing body in the world and they don't licence anything that doesn't work.

It's widely used by doctors throughout the world, doctors in private practice that is. I work with doctors; some of my best friends are doctors. I've treated an awful lot of doctors and their families for their own personal health problems over the years so you see I like doctors really. Most of the time it's not doctors that are at fault but the so-called healthcare system that they are trapped in. Most doctors learn of me and of my work when I cure their patients or I'm recommended by one of their colleagues that has already been to see me.

If a doctor has a personal health problem and they can't find the answer themselves then they have to look elsewhere, so they come to people like me. There are a lot of unhealthy doctors out there you know! Many doctors are worse than their patients ...if the public only knew! Doctors are only human they get sick just like everyone else. In fact according to an American poll doctors die on average 20 years younger than the rest of the population and they have one of the highest suicide rates and occurrences of drink related problems of professional people.

Why does that not surprise me!

WHY DOCTORS DON'T MAKE YOU HEALTHY.

I have no problem with most doctors, it's just that their time and budgets could be better spent. If doctors knew how to treat people with this technology then they'd cure 80% or more of their patients overnight and the money they would have wasted on unnecessary drugs could be put to better use. So!...I hear you ask...if what I say is true then why are doctors not being taught this method of treatment in medical schools?. For the very simple reason that most medical schools are either **directly** or **indirectly** subsidised, financed and/or supported by drug companies and as I've already said it's not in any drug companies **business** interest to promote a method of healthcare that makes people healthy without drugs.

Most of the time the best you are going to get as a patient is medication to **relieve** the problem then you have to buy some more next week when the problem comes back again. Wouldn't it be better for a patient if we could find what was causing their headache and other health problems, so that when they avoided a particular food they wouldn't experience the problem?

*Ah!...But what if it's **not** food that's causing the headache or other problems?*

In my experience food intolerance is a **major** cause of headaches and most other general everyday health problems. I've carried out thousands of scans over the last ten years and I've seen thousands of people becoming healthy as a result. In my opinion food intolerance testing should always be considered **before** any other form of treatment. If the problem still exists a few months later then that is the time to carry out other tests. But if they gave this a chance to work first then they would find that most general health problems disappeared within a month or so.

So why don't doctors talk about Food Intolerance with their patients?

Most of them don't even know it exists, they are not taught this at medical school so how could they know. So if they don't know about it how can they inform their patients? And for many doctors if they haven't been taught it then there not interested anyway. They prefer to plod along doing what they've been trained to do and keep their head in the sand whilst writing out thousands of useless and costly prescriptions.

I'm not so sure that their bosses would allow them to use this treatment anyway as they have very strict rules on what doctors can and can't do. Also many of the big wigs that run the medical profession will probably have shares or other interests in drug companies, so **why** would they want to change anything?
When you think about it in fairness to the public they serve and that employs them and in order to ensure that they are seen to be whiter than white in their decision making, they should be made to dispose of such financial and other interests prior to being appointed to these highly paid management positions. MPs have to declare their interests, so why not these people also?

Chapter **4**

THE FOUNDATION FOR INTEGRATED MEDICINE

Somebody once said to me:

"Prince Charles is into Alternative Medicine, why don't you write to him."

So I did!…in January 2001.

Here's a shortened version of the letter:

Monday 8th January 2001

Email: **intolerance@healthscan.co.uk**

Dear Prince Charles,

I know you have a keen interest in Alternative Medicine and that you support it through your association with The Foundation for Integrated Medicine. I write in the hope that you might consider supporting the work that I do in the field of Food Intolerance.
As you will see from the enclosed, the results of a **'single'** food intolerance test are quite dramatic. Please also try and find time to look at my website: www.healthscan.co.uk I know you will find it very interesting and informative.

Basically, as I am sure you know there is a great resistance in conventional medicine to anything that eliminates the need for drugs. The fact that such alternatives actually work is of no consequence. If drug companies were to cure people then they would go out of business, so from a business point of view why would they want to make people healthy? They have not become the biggest companies in the world by making people healthy.

With this technology the cost of drugs to the Health Service could be cut by 50% or more overnight, people would become healthy and the money saved could be put to better use. The public has a right to know that there are alternatives when it comes to being healthy. With your help maybe we can break down the in-depth resistance of the medical establishment to such change.

I look forward to hearing from you.

Regards,

Gerard Kielty I.R.B; I.D.E .

It seems Prince Charles is President of: 'The Foundation for Integrated Medicine' as you can see from the letter overleaf when his secretary replied and suggested that I contact the foundation direct.

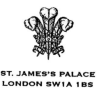

ST. JAMES'S PALACE
LONDON SW1A 1BS

From: The Deputy Private Secretary to HRH The Prince of Wales

16th January 2001

The Prince of Wales has asked me to thank you for your letter of 8th January enclosing information about the work you do in the field of food intolerance testing. His Royal Highness has suggested that you might like to contact the Chief Executive of The Foundation for Integrated Medicine of which he is President. The Foundation's details are shown below:-

Michael Fox Esq
Chief Executive
The Foundation for Integrated Medicine
International House
59 Compton Road
London N1 2YT

In the meantime I know The Prince of Wales would wish me to thank you for your kindness in having taken the trouble to write and to send you his best wishes.

Mark Bolland

Gerard Kielty Esq IRB IDE

Figure 4: Letter from the Deputy Private Secretary of HRH The Prince of Wales.

So I wrote to them and sent loads of testimonial letters/editorials/CD's etc:

Thursday 25th January 2001

Email: intolerance@healthscan.co.uk

Dear Mr Fox,

Having looked at my work in the field of Food Intolerance HRH Prince Charles the Prince of Wales has requested that I contact you. Should you wish to confirm this then please telephone his private secretary Mr Mark Bolland at St. James's Palace.

You will clearly see from the enclosed material just how effective my work is. Please also spare a little time to view my website at www.healthscan.co.uk as you will find it full of very interesting information on food intolerance.

I will let the enclosed speak for it self, only to say that I very much look forward to meeting with you with a view to jointly promoting my work through the foundation.

Regards,

GERARD KIELTY I.R.B; I.D.E.

A month later I had heard nothing so I wrote to Mr Fox again.

Within a few days I received a phone call from Patricia Darnell manager of their Research and Development department telling me that Mr Fox was on holiday and that she would ensure that he was given my package upon his return. We had a good lengthy chat and she seemed quite interested and impressed with my work but from what I could make of it the foundation don't actually do much apart from gather information on Alternative Health and formulate it in some way before passing it onward and upward to the powers that be.

Mr Fox did write to me upon his return from holiday.

Full text of his letter is on the next page.

For copyright reasons the original letter cannot be shown.
But the full text of the letter is as follows

THE FOUNDATION FOR INTEGRATED MEDICINE

26th February 2001

Dear Mr Kielty,

Thank you for your letter of 19th February and enclosures.

I understand that Patricia Darnell, Research and Development Manager, has spoken to you about the Foundations objectives and current projects. Whilst we are unable to assist you on this occasion, Patricia will investigate other areas of potential over the next few months.

Please find enclosed some information on the Foundation.

Yours sincerely,

Michael Fox
Chief Executive.

Figure 5: Letter from the Foundation for Integrated Medicine

So, that was the letter I received from Chief Executive Mr Michael Fox dated 26th February 2001 stating that Patricia would investigate other areas of potential over the next few months.

What other areas of potential? And why try to stall me?

Am I missing something here or are these people not set up to **promote** alternative medicine when and where possible? I've just sent these people masses of proof that I cure over fifty different health problems without the need for drugs and all I get back is a **Dear John** letter. A letter that is basically saying **please go away** and leave us to our **tax-free** charitable status cushy little jobs. The only reason I got a reply in the first place signed by the Chief Executive was that I was pointed in there direction by Prince Charles.

Now some five years later I'm still waiting for Patricia to get back to me with exciting news of **other areas of potential**.
If I can't get things moving with an introduction from Prince Charles then I don't hold out much hope for other people contacting the foundation in the future.

I guess it must be **'THE ESTABLISHMENT'S'** way of keeping an eye on what's going on out here in the world of Alternative Medicine. Anyway look on the bright side the foundation gets a nice tax-free grant for their troubles from the Kings Fund (whatever that is) so I guess they're happy enough. Other letters from world leaders are shown in Appendix 2. Suffice it here to say they were very similar in their style and approach to the subject.

Chapter **5**

THE OPPOSITION

Some years back a consultant paediatrician referred several children to me for treatment from a major teaching hospital on the South coast of England and they all made incredible recoveries. She had heard about my work initially because I had cured one of her patients. This child was about eight years old and from birth she had I.B.S. coughed continuously, was considerably underweight, physically sick all the time and very irritable. She was admitted to hospital on a regular basis and all they could offer her was a bedside drip, they had been treating her for years. They just didn't know what to do with her.

Eventually her mother brought her to see me, I carried out a food intolerance test and she became a **normal healthy child** within a few months.

There's a testimonial letter from her mother later in the book.

Anyway, the point I'm making is that the hospital managers found out about the consultant sending children to me for food intolerance testing and they threatened to terminate her contract if she sent anymore. The fact that I actually made the children **healthy** was totally irrelevant to them.

I offered to teach the consultant how to use this scanner so that she could get one into the hospital and treat the children herself. She was keen but unfortunately the powers that be were not, so that was the end of that. This was just one of **many** examples of rejection by the medical world over the years. You will read of many more later in this book. People often say it must be very frustrating for me to have a scanning system that makes people healthy and to get rejected like that. I'm well used to the medical profession not wanting to know

Okay!...I've proved it makes people healthy so **why** *are they not interested?*

Well....I think one reason is that the higher people go **up** the management ladder the **less** they want to...or are **allowed** to make decisions.

But why? ...I hear you say.

Because it's far safer to leave things as they are than to risk making a decision. If you make a **bad** decision when your running a hospital and/or government department and your on a salary of say £140,000 a year or more then you have a long way to fall. So!...the safest way is to leave things as they are. That way you continue to rake in your **fat salary** and you don't risk upsetting anybody.

*But why you say would they not want this equipment when it has been **proven** to make people healthy...surely the patients come first?*

I guess it's because the system as it is makes billions of pounds each and every year and provides large salaries for drug company executives and those in power.

Pharmaceutical companies make **huge** profits from selling drugs and governments rake in colossal sums from taxes **on** drugs. It works very nicely! So everyone's happy apart from the patient that is, who spends a lot of money on long-term medication and continues to suffer. I'll leave you to make your own decision as to whose pockets are being lined. Hopefully public opinion will eventually force governments to act and then something will have to be done. The crazy thing is if politicians really cared about the people they represented and actually changed the system then my bet is that they would make more money by having a country full of healthy people. Firstly!...We wouldn't need nearly as many hospital beds and doctors as we do now, so billions of pounds would be saved each and every year. There would also be millions more people **in** work instead of sitting at home and living off sickness benefit. These new healthy people would then be paying taxes **into** the system and not taking money **from** the system. And that's just the tip of the iceberg, I'm sure there must be a vast number of other ways that both the government and the public would benefit.

You may well say that all the decision makers in health and government can't be the same, surely there are some that would want to do the right thing where the public are concerned. Yes!...I have no doubt that there are some with good intentions but there's this huge brick wall out there called

'THE ESTABLISHMENT'

It's been around for a **very** long time and it's **very** well protected. And I can assure you that it takes more than a single individual or a group of do-gooders to knock that wall down.

Again you might ask: *Is it that the people at the top just don't believe you or that they think it can't possibly work?*

These people are not fools. They know exactly what the score is. They know that if they took too much of an interest in this technology then they would have to incorporate it into the public healthcare system; **or** come up with a convincing explanation to the public as to why they didn't. It's called **progress** and there are many people out there in the world of medicine that would rather turn a blind eye to it for their own selfish reasons. But one thing they can never argue with are results and I get them all the time.

My father used to say:
"There are none as blind as those that **will not** see."

How true!

I travel the world a great deal in my work and wherever I go I'm always very busy. But I'd be totally swamped with patients if the greater majority of people throughout the world knew of my work and the results I get. But for that to happen I need to get to the masses. Simply scanning a person or doing occasional radio and TV interviews or relying on recommendations and editorials will never get the word out to any great extent. It's just too big a world out there so that's why I've written this book.

You may say: '*Why don't you advertise on the radio or TV or in the national press, you could get to a lot of people that way.*'

Tried it!...I can't get a licence to advertise and secondly have you seen the cost of advertising on national radio or television and in the national newspapers?...they're talking telephone numbers. It's only the **drug companies** that can afford those prices. Even if I were to be granted a licence, such a high cost of advertising would push my scanning fees through the roof. Thus leaving only the rich to benefit from this treatment. To advertise anything medical on TV/radio or in the national press you're application has to be vetted by a **medical** committee to see if you can be granted a licence, so there lies another problem.

The committee is made up of doctors and people from **within** that big brick wall and they have **no intention** of letting people like me in.   So you go round in ever decreasing circles and get nowhere as usual. It's just **THE ESTABLISHMENT** protecting itself once again with its well tested and finely tuned self-defence mechanism.

You've never seen an Alternative Health Therapist advertising on television...have you?

All you see on TV are drugs promoted by the big boys.
Almost every advertising break has at least one drug for sale sometimes two or three. They have it all to themselves, after all they've got the money and no doubt they look after the right people... **if** you know what I mean. It would be interesting to check just how many ex-Health Ministers and/or other government ministers or management of the NHS were given a seat on the board of drug companies over the past 50 years or so and I wonder also just how many brown envelopes may have changed hands along the way.
Do you really think that if I discovered how to run a car on water that I'd have any chance of marketing it? There are just too many powerful people out there making vast sums of money from oil.
I'd have no chance...Would I?

Well it's the same with 'Drugs' and the health business.

I've written to two or three different Health Ministers and a few Prime Ministers over the years telling them of my work and offering to carryout **FREE** clinical trials in hospitals in order to prove it's effectiveness beyond doubt. I didn't get a single reply (apart from Tony Blair, see Appendix 2). It seems I was wrong to assume that they would be interested.

WHY DOCTORS DON'T MAKE YOU HEALTHY.

I can only come to the conclusion therefore that they are all part of the same set-up and it's all a big game to them. I suppose the system as it is generates vast sums of money every year in taxes and I guess there's no way they want to risk changing that.

As I said before if people got better the government would save billions of pounds every year by not having to pay out for hospitals and doctors and unnecessary drugs and sickness claims. But to make such far-reaching changes to a monster such as the NHS would upset a lot of **very powerful** people and I don't think that would go down too well within The Establishment.

There are after all election funds to consider.

Maybe once you have read this book you would be kind enough to email your Prime Minister, President or Health Minister and ask them why you are not being allowed to have this scanning system in your hospitals when it has been proven to cure most everyday health problems without drugs. Please send me a copy of their reply…I would be most interested.

My email address is: intolerance@healthscan.co.uk

I would very much welcome the chance to ask the PM or Health Minister that and many other questions 'live' on TV if anyone is prepared to produce such a programme.

I have a theory and it's only a theory. I have no way of proving it one way or the other but another reason that governments around the world don't want to change anything is possibly that as the system is at the moment most people die at around 60 or 70 years of age…give or take a few years. And for most of our lives we buy drugs in one form or another just to get by from day-to-day and governments all over the world make a great deal of money from the tax we pay on those drugs. In my opinion it is just conceivable that the use of these drugs cause their own long-term health problems and possibly kill us off years before we would have died anyway. Now! Think about this…until we get to 60 for women and 65 for men we pay money **to** the government in the form of income tax and after that **they** pay us in the form of a pension. So therefore it's obviously not in the government's financial interest that we should live too long after our retirement age.

Well!...Heavy or not it does make you think!...Hold on I have a report here somewhere.

This was taken from BBC Ceefax on Tuesday 17th July 2001.
It reads:
A Tobacco company commissioned an internal report on their industry in Czechoslovakia and presented it to the government.
It showed that premature deaths of smokers left the government $100 million **better off** in 1999 with regard to healthcare and pensions.

So!...The government actually saved **$100 million** in 'ONE YEAR' from the premature deaths of smokers by **not** having to care for them in hospitals and by **not** having to pay them a pension.

Plus!

The government made a vast amount of revenue from the tax the poor souls paid on the cigarettes in the first place. Now just think about it: if Czechoslovakia can save **$100 million a year** in that way how much do you think the UK government or the US government saves through **premature** deaths each and every year? And I don't just mean tobacco related deaths!

Is that how governments see us when we're ill and elderly...as a financial liability?

Yeah!…I know!…Interesting don't you think? I doubt if any country could afford to be **top heavy** with pensioners. But as I say it's only a theory, I don't know one way or the other but when they don't even reply to my letters which I sent with testimonial letters and masses of researched editorials from national newspapers…plus loads of other information it does make you wonder just what **is** going on up there in those great corridor's of power.

Another option:
What about **Health Insurance** companies? They'd be good to approach; it would save them a fortune as they wouldn't have to keep **paying out** for expensive tests for their members. And what about the various charity organisations that are set up to promote research into Eczema and Migraine etc. Surely they'd be interested in my work? Been there!…Read the book!…Seen the video!…They all have their own little (tax free) empires running and there making a nice **fat** living!…So the **last** thing they would want is change.

But surely (you say) *they are there to help people find a cure isn't that **why** they were set up in the first place?*

Well it would be nice to think so! But I've run clinical trials for lots of these groups over the years and I've proved that my scanning works and still nothing happens.

But why not? (you say) *if you're making people better…surely that's what they want isn't it?*

Well, I used to think that too but just stop for a moment and think about it from their point of view. You're a director of a large charity or other organisation set up to promote good health in one field or another and you've got say 80,000 members or more.

Each of these members is paying you say £20 (or more) a year in membership fees and you are probably getting a hefty government grant as well. In addition these types of company are often registered charities so you don't have to pay tax. Your charity also earns a nice little income each year from selling thousands of so-called **'helpful'** books and other such products to your members. Plus they get considerable revenue from people advertising in their literature. Then this guy from Health Scan comes along with a computer that can make your members better! **Holy smoke!** Do you really want to allow him into your organisation! Hey!…that's the last thing you'd want. If he started making your members better you'd go out of business.

Oh!…And as far as the Health Insurance Companies are concerned you can be very sure indeed that they **take in** in premiums far more than they **pay out** in claims otherwise they wouldn't be there in the first place. Its **fear** of ill health that makes people take out insurance. So they wouldn't want to promote a computerised scanning system that could wipe out 80% of health problems would they!

***

Yes!…I can see it now!…drug companies and governments throughout the world will do all they can to assure the public that this technology is nonsense; they'll come up with every trick in the book in order to fight it.

Vegetarian Groups!…Migraine organisations!…Eczema and dozens of other such organisations will all be up in arms. But the public are not stupid, once they've read this book and tried the diet that I've recommended for two months or so they'll see the results for themselves and be able to make up their own minds.

Doctors from time to time come up with the same old argument that Alternative Medicine isn't real medicine. Well if they care to look back before the good old days of **'Conventional Medicine'** they will see that there were other ways of treating the sick. So therefore conventional medicine could also be said to be alternative.

❖ Text was written as far back as 1250BC on healthcare treatments with electric eels.

❖ Dr William Gilbert wrote a book on electricity and the body in the 1600's.

❖ In 1752 Johann Schaeffer wrote a book on Electrical Medicine.

❖ 1830. Carlo Matteucci showed how Electrical Medicine could regenerate body tissue.

❖ In 1858 Dr Francis used Electrical Medicine to relieve dental pain.

So let's not hear talk about **'Alternative'** medicine being inferior all forms of medicine are alternative to one another. Just because alternative treatments and therapies are different from conventional medicine it doesn't make them any less effective, in fact in many cases such as in my work it makes them **more** effective.

The best way to judge any form of medicine is by results.

PART 2

FRUIT AND

VEGETABLES;

THE KILLER FOODS

Chapter **6**

SO WHAT FOODS GENERALLY CAUSE THE MOST HEALTH PROBLEMS?

Vegetables!

Yes!…Vegetables!

"But vegetables are good for me!" I hear you shout.

Q: Who told you that vegetables are good for you?

A: We were brought up to believe it, it's pumped into us over the years. Everything we read and see in books and on television tells us that vegetables are **'good'** for us. We were all brainwashed into believing that vegetables were good for us even before we could read.

Q: Who told you as a child that vegetables were good for you?

A: *"My mum, I suppose!"*

Exactly!…And who told your mum?

And therein lies the problem!…This advice has been handed down over generations just like doctors teach doctors; mums and dad's teach their kids. But I'm the first person to check what these drugs are doing to **your** brain. Foods and other things need to be checked if you're putting them into your body to ensure that they are not giving your brain a problem. As you now know everything you put into your body **is** a drug **to** your brain and it'll have a positive or a negative effect **on** your brain.

Don't get me wrong I have nothing against vegetables. It's just that they are the group of foods that in my experience cause the most health problems. If vegetables were all they are cracked up to be then vegetarians would stand out from the crowd as looking super healthy! Do they?

Don't let it worry you though not all vegetables are bad, just different vegetables to different people.

Why are vegetables so bad?

Don't know!...They just are!...As I said before, heroin grows in the ground, well so does a lettuce. They are both drugs, the only difference is that they each give off their own **unique** electrical signal and that's what arrives at our brain.

Oh!...And Herbs and Spices are just as bad by the way.

Yes!...They're just as bad as vegetables, if not worse!

Well!...When you think about it they are vegetables, they grow in the ground just the same as conventional vegetables do.

Let me ask you a question.

Would you walk into the middle of the woods and pick some weird plant and eat it?

No!...Of course you wouldn't.

Well that's all a herb is, a weird plant!
Somebody has pulled it from the ground and stuck it in a fancy jar and told you it's good for you!...**Is it?**...How would they know? It might well poison your brain...nobody knows or really cares just so long as you buy it.

"But I like herbs and spices, I feel good when I eat them." ...you reply.

Yes!...and drug addicts feel good when they take drugs! Surely it makes sense to **check** where possible just what these things are doing to your brain if and when you eat them.
We have the technology so why not use it?

"But don't you eat vegetables?" ...many of you will be asking.

No!...Not really, I might have the odd one or two here and there if I'm eating out from time to time but even then I usually leave most of them on the plate. Although I do eat potatoes in one form or another on a fairly regular basis I suppose. I was never brought up with having to eat vegetables; my parents took the attitude that if I didn't want them then leave them and go hungry. I came from a big family and my ten brothers and sisters were the same, none of us ate much in the way of vegetables and none of us have ever suffered with **Asthma!**...or **Eczema!**...or anything else of much consequence in the way of health problems.
When you think about it most kids don't like vegetables anyway...do they!

I've had mothers break down in tears when they came to realise how they'd been poisoning their children by forcing them to eat vegetables. In my opinion if kids had a food intolerance test once a year from the age of 5 when they start at primary school then 80% of health problems would never materialise in the first place.

As I said earlier we tune our cars up every year to keep them running properly, so why don't we do the same with our brain? The scanning system I use is doing just that, it's a kind of **'Tune up'** machine for the brain.

The Top Ten Most Troublesome Foods

1. MINT (IT'S IN YOUR TOOTHPASTE)

2. YEAST (ALSO IN BEER/WINE/CHAMPAGNE)

3. SUGAR (ALSO IN CHOCOLATE.....SORRY!)

4. WHEAT (PASTA/SPAGHETTI/BISCUITS)

5. ALL FRUIT (DRINKING/EATING/DRIED)

6. SALT (DO NOT ADD TO FOOD)

7. POTATOES (ALSO CRISPS AND VODKA)

8. TOMATOES (ALSO KETCHUP)

9. MUSHROOMS (THESE ARE A YEAST FUNGUS)

10. CHEESE (ALL FORMS)

Chapter 7

MINT!
A MAJOR CAUSE OF HEALTH
PROBLEMS

Over the years I have found **mint** to be a major cause of health problems and it's in the toothpaste we use each and every day.

Toothpaste!...But **'everyone'** *uses toothpaste!* I hear you shout.

Yes!...And as I have proved thousands of times that's one of the main reasons why most people are unhealthy!

But we don't swallow toothpaste!

We don't have to swallow it for it to affect our brain, it's absorbed through the sublingual glands under our tongue and it hits our brain within a fraction of a second of us putting the brush in our mouth.

(See **YOUR DIET TO GOOD HEALTH** on Page 69 for toothpaste advice)

In my experience mint is one of the worst drugs our brain has to endure and my work over the years has clearly shown it to be a major factor in causing serious health problems. If you think about it most supermarket checkouts and other retail outlets such as petrol filling stations and newsagents have a vast array of mint products on display right next to the till. This is the one place in the store that you are most likely to buy on impulse; it's also a place that people often have to queue. When at this point young children faced with an array of sweets will ask for some. More often than not it's mints that mum or dad will choose believing them to be healthier for their child than conventional sweets.

When I scan a person I am more than surprised if their **not** intolerant to spearmint and/or peppermint. About 95% of the ten thousand or so patients I've scanned **were** intolerant to one or both of them.

When you are following **YOUR DIET TO GOOD HEALTH** you must stop using mint toothpaste, mint mouthwash, mint chewing gum and mint sweets.

So, how has this situation come about? I think that we've just become intolerant to mint because we put it into our mouth every day of our lives on the end of a toothbrush. But I reckon that if people stopped using mint toothpaste there would be a major worldwide collapse of pharmaceutical companies. The thing I don't understand though is if I've found such a link between mint and ill health why have the drug companies not also found it?

I'll leave you to make up your own mind on that one!

Note:
Do not be surprised if your children cannot settle after putting them to bed, or they have nightmares or wet the bed. This is typical of what can happen when the brain has just been poisoned. Schoolwork will also suffer through lack of concentration and/or other health problems quiet possibly caused by mint in toothpaste.

Chapter **8**

YEAST AND SUGAR THE BIGGEST CAUSES OF HEALTH PROBLEMS!

First, a few facts about yeast:

Yeast is a living fungus it's what we call phlegm or mucus.
We all have yeast in our body. It's passed on in the womb.
Yeast is one of the few things in our body that is **not** controlled by our brain.
Yeast breathes **in** Oxygen and breaths **out** Carbon Dioxide just as we do, this process is called fermentation.
Yeast is by far the biggest cause of health problems in the body.
I would say that 70% **or more** of the people I've scanned had a yeast problem of one sort or another.
Yeast affects all regions of the body, it's a living fungus.
Yeast lives wherever it chooses too, anywhere **in** or **on** the body.
Yeast is a major cause of **Asthma**.
Yeast is a major cause of **Bloated Stomach** and **Irritable Bowel**.
Yeast in the diet has two basic forms: **Bakers Yeast & Brewers Yeast**.
Yeast is the sole cause of **Colic** in babies. You would think that the medical profession would have worked that one out by now.
Yeast blocks the Eustachian tube's that run from the back of our throat to the inner ear. Their sole purpose is to ventilate the inner ear (behind the eardrum) with oxygen. When these tubes block up it causes conditions such as **Tinnitus** (ringing in the ear) **Dizziness** and **Infection**.
Yeast is the sole cause of **Thrush**.

Yeast is the sole cause of **Athletes Foot**.
Yeast is the sole cause of **Hiatus Hernia**.
Yeast is a major cause of **Hay Fever**.
(According to the B.B.C. website 9 million people in the UK suffer with Hay Fever and I cure it with a 'single' scan!)
Yeast is a major cause of **Mouth Ulcers**.
Yeast is a major cause of **Stomach Ulcers**.
A Mushroom is a yeast fungus.
Penicillin is a yeast fungus.
Antibiotics are a yeast fungus; these are mostly made of Penicillin.
Cataracts that grow across the surface of the eyeball are a yeast fungus.

The only way to bring yeast under control is to **STOP** putting it into your body (for six months or so) and to **STOP** feeding the yeast that's already in your body.

And what does yeast live on?

SUGAR!

Fruit is a major cause of health problems!

Yes!…You did read it right!
'Fruit' is a major cause of health problems.

Why?

Because fruit is full of sugar!
The sugar is called **Fructose!**…and guess what!…yeast love it.

'AN APPLE A DAY KEEPS THE DOCTOR AWAY'

To the contrary…It brings him much closer!

It would not surprise me to learn that drug companies financed the promotion of that slogan many years ago. Even Adam & Eve in the Garden of Eden were told **NOT** to eat the apple!...*And you know who told them!*

As I mentioned earlier I'm one of 11 children, we were not brought up on fruit. We thought ourselves lucky if we got an orange in our Xmas stocking or for our birthday. Not one of us has ever suffered with Asthma / Eczema / I.B.S. etc. Apart from the odd broken bone here and there playing sport we all had a very healthy childhood. My point is that you do not need fruit to be healthy! In fact I have cured thousands of people by getting them **off** fruit!

Imagine the scenario:
You're lying in a hospital bed suffering with Asthma… I.B.S. or any other yeast complaint and your loving visitors bring you fruit!

Yeah!...Just what you need!

If you want to do a simple yeast test then spit a little phlegm into a glass of cold water immediately upon waking in the morning. Keep the glass stationary and check it a few hours later, if your spit has grown long stringy tentacles then you have very active yeast in your body. I would not say that this test is 100% accurate but it does give you a pretty good indication of your yeast condition. All the answers you need to beat yeast will be found in the next chapter.

Chapter **9**

YOUR DIET TO GOOD HEALTH

A couple of words that come up time after time when doctors give dietary advice to their patients are **'Balanced diet.'** What they fail to realise is that each and every patient is an individual **(we all have a unique brain)** and each and every food **(drug)** will affect their brain in its own way. Every patient is an individual and should be treated as such. Balanced diets do not cater for the individual. My diet below advises on what foods to avoid rather than what foods to eat.

This diet is recommended for everyone *(apart from children younger than 4 years old)* to try for a minimum of six months although nine months to a year would be even more beneficial.

You will find that within a few months many if not all of your health problems will have disappeared or will be a great deal better. The most important thing you have to remember is **not** to rush the changes to your diet. Wean off the foods listed below that you are currently eating on a regular basis *(i.e. at least once a week)* this includes your toothpaste. Do not make the changes too fast or you could get worse before you get better. The reason is that foods and mint in toothpaste are drugs to your brain and if you come off troublesome **drugs** too quickly then you may well experience what is known as **'COLD TURKEY.'** Your brain will be craving the drugs **(fix)** that it was used to and it could then be thrown into an even more confused state than it is currently in. It has taken a lifetime to get your chemistry into its current state so give yourself a month or two to change it.

WHY DOCTORS DON'T MAKE YOU HEALTHY.

After all that you've read in this book there may still be one or two of you that will question as to how you can possibly be healthy without fruit and vegetables. To the contrary and as I have proved thousands of times a great deal of your current health problems are being **caused** by them. Apart from having a food intolerance test carried out the only way you will ever know for sure if these foods are a problem is to come off them and watch the results.

As I mentioned above the following diet is not forever, if you wish to go back onto the foods in six months or so then that's fine but I would advise staying off them for nine months to a year. Normally when patients return to eating previously troublesome foods the foods have ceased to be a problem. This is probably because the brain has had a chance to recover and is now in a better state to handle them. It is rare that a food continues to cause trouble, once it has been removed from the diet for six months or so it's normally acceptable once more. Those of you that follow my advice will reap the rewards in due course, please don't forget to take a few minutes once you've become healthy to write a testimonial letter and send it to me via email:

intolerance@healthscan.co.uk

Every testimonial letter is another step forward, another step nearer the day that this computerised scanning will be made available at your local hospital or GP surgery. Without testimonial letters there is no evidence of the effectiveness of this technology. Also if we are to ensure that our children and grandchildren do not continue to suffer unnecessarily at the hands of drug companies then do try to support me in whatever way you can through radio/television newspaper editorials and the media in general.

One should avoid **SUGAR** and **YEAST** based products, these include:

Fruit... Fruit drinks and dried fruits of all kinds.
Sugared bottled/canned drinks also **diet** drinks as these contain artificial sugars.
Avoid all **artificial** sweeteners in tea and coffee.
Do not drink Wine / Beer / Champagne or Cider as these contain yeast and fruit sugars.
If you want a drink then have a Gin, Brandy or Whisky but don't put a tonic or any other sweet mixer with it. Don't drink Rum as this is sugar based and don't drink Vodka as this is made from potatoes which turn into sugar.

Before we go any further I will be the first to admit that you cannot totally avoid **sugar!** Just do your best without becoming a complete pain in the butt to those around you. Your current cravings for sugar and other foods will slowly decrease over the next few months as you start to become healthy. It's like a drink to an alcoholic or a cigarette to a smoker, you will slowly start to feel better by not having too much of these things and as a result you will want less of them.

Do not drink **cows milk** (skimmed or otherwise) as it contains a sugar called lactose. You may drink (unsweetened) **Soya milk** or **goat's milk** as these do not contain sugar.

Do not eat **yoghurt** as this will often contain **sugar** based items. It will definitely always contain **live bacteria** and probably **yeast** and you do not want these in your body.

Avoid **sugar** based breakfast cereals and use the right milk.

No **jam, marmalade** or **honey** as these all contain sugar.

WHY DOCTORS DON'T MAKE YOU HEALTHY.

A food item may often show on the label that there are **no added sugars**, be careful as it may already contain sugar and they just haven't added any!

No **cheese** of any description (including goat's cheese) as it contains yeast!

No **spreads** that contain yeast.

If when reading this book you feel that you have a big yeast problem then it would be wise to avoid **wheat** for four months or so as it's a major carbohydrate and as such it turns into sugar in your body. The other carbohydrates you must also avoid in this respect are **rice, potatoes, rye, corn** and **oats**.
If however you feel that your yeast problem may only be minor then leave wheat, rice and potatoes alone and eat only a little of rye bread (yeast free) corn and oats.

Don't eat **pastries** or things that rise up when cooked as these will generally contain yeast *(i.e. bases of pizzas)*

No **chocolate** or **drinking chocolate** as these contain sugar.
(I know ladies...sorry but it's the only way to get healthy, I promise it will be worth it)

Don't use **wine** in cooking.

No sweet and sour meals at your Chinese restaurant, the sweet part is **honey**.

Drink **still** not carbonated water. (Great with your Gin!)
(Keep your liquid intake low if you want to lose weight, see WEIGHT on Page 155)

Eggs seem to suit most people and there's a lot you can make with them.

Forget convention with breakfast, dinner and tea.
Eat the **right things** at any time of the day or night.
Have a cold chicken leg for breakfast or something left over from last night's dinner.

Buy a large range of **Homeopathic** toothpastes, say 8 or 10 different flavours and each time you pick up your toothbrush pick up a different tube of toothpaste. Do not use the same toothpaste on a daily basis; rotate your toothpaste flavours each time you brush your teeth. In this way there is less chance of any flavour becoming a problem to your brain.

When eating, eat slowly, and eat small meals or snacks during the day as opposed to one or two big main meals. If you're used to eating a great deal of food then slowly try and reduce the volume of food you put into your body. You will find that as you get healthier over the next few weeks and months you will want less and less food.

Again I will remind you to avoid all **current** vegetables when possible for at least 6 months or better still up to 9 months.
(If you want the occasional 'new' vegetable then that's okay... but don't eat them on a regular basis)
If you have any current cravings for foods then come off them slowly as they are almost certainly causing problems in your brain. Take a daily multi **Vitamin & Mineral** tablet and don't be frightened to get out and take at least a little exercise once you start to feel better.

Come off **ALL** mint products, especially toothpaste.

Chapter **10**

SALT

❖ Salt conducts **ELECTRICITY** in the Nervous System.
❖ It makes a **SMALL** headache into a **BIG** headache.
❖ It makes a **SMALL** skin problem into a **BIG** skin problem.

The good signals coming from your brain don't need any help so don't make the bad ones worse. Remember: You only have to put salt onto a cut to know how much it upsets your brain.
Your brain tells you it doesn't like salt by sending out a signal called pain.

Don't eat foods regularly that are covered with salt.
(i.e.: Crisps/peanuts)

Yes!...We know that your body needs salt but you will find that it gets more than enough naturally from foods. Don't add it when you are cooking or when the food is on your plate. When you eat out in a restaurant and there's salt in your food then eat it but don't order foods that you know are rich in salt. If you eat Chinese food more than once a month then ask them to cook your meal without Monosodium Glutamate. This is a salt that they use in Chinese cooking and it will cause a lot of problems for those who have it on a regular basis.

Chapter **11**

GENERAL ADVICE

Don't take any non-prescribed remedies that you have bought in a Chemist or Health Food shop. You will not need any remedy to recover, you will get better by **not** putting things into your body and simply letting your brain do the job it was designed to do, the job of running your body efficiently. Avoid anything your doctor has not prescribed.

Please ensure that you talk to your doctor before coming off prescribed medication.

Do remember that this is not **ALLERGY** advice but **FOOD INTOLERANCE** advice. These two things are totally different as you can be allergic to things you are not intolerant to and visa-versa. If you're not sure of your allergies then check with your doctor.

Do not bath in Essential Oils or rub them into your skin as these are made from herbs.

Do not burn strong smelling candles on a regular basis.

Remember it doesn't matter how an item gets into your body you can inhale it/inject it/absorb it through your skin or eat or drink it. Whichever way it gets into your body it will always end up acting as a drug to your brain.

Wear gloves if you are handling foods that you should not be eating.

WHY DOCTORS DON'T MAKE YOU HEALTHY.

I have never yet had to test for the effects of makeup in order to make people healthy.

Be aware of things you're eating and drinking on a regular basis and change them around from time to time. Even if you feel good on them, remember drug addicts feel **good** on drugs!

Do not cook with the same oil all the time.

Don't eat or drink strong flavoured things too often. (i.e. Curry or Whisky) If they're giving your taste buds a shock then what might they be doing to your brain?

Whether you have current health problems or not you will feel the benefit of putting a little eye ointment/cream into your eyes every now and again. Pop into your local chemist shop/pharmacy and buy some eye ointment. Buy a tube of **ointment** and not **eye drops** as it will lubricate better and stay in your eyes longer than a liquid.

If you wear contact lenses I have no way of knowing if the cream will damage the material of the lens. I don't for one-minute think that it will but I don't know for sure. Put a little cream into your eyes a few times a week last thing at night before you jump into bed. You'll find that the extra eye lubrication feels great and reduces eye sensitivity. It also kills yeast fungus that loves to live in and around the eye socket. After a few months stop using the ointment on a regular basis only use it occasionally as you feel you need it. Store your ointment in the fridge to keep it fresh.

WARNING:
**DO NOT SHARE YOUR TUBE OF OINTMENT
WITH OTHERS AS YOU MAY CROSS INFECT EYES**

Always try and buy **'IMPREGNATED NASAL TISSUES'** these will be impregnated with substances such as **Balm** and **Lanolin** that give the tissue a velvet like touch and cut down dramatically on the dust given off. Whether a person has respiratory problems or not it is a good idea to cut down on the paper dust that enters our body when we use a normal tissue on our nose. If you pull a tissue from its box and hold it up to a ray of sunlight you will see a huge cloud of paper dust.

When you are using a tissue you are inhaling this dust through your mouth and nose and it will irritate sensitive nerve endings in your body, especially those in your respiratory tract.

IMPREGNATED TISSUES ARE 'ESSENTIAL' FOR THOSE SUFFERING WITH RESPIRATORY, EYE OR NASAL PROBLEMS OF ANY KIND.

Here's another of my cynical theories for your consideration:
If tissue manufacturers wished to increase sales then it would make sense to make them as dusty as possible. Because the more dust that goes up your nose the more you sneeze and the more you sneeze the more tissues you need.

If your fingernails are a mess from biting and/or picking them *(this is a nervous condition often caused by eating the wrong foods)* then buy yourself a **nail clipper** and a **nail file** *(emery board)* and **use** them! Keep them handy and tidy up those loose ends of skin and nail on a regular basis. As you get your foods sorted over the next few months and take your vitamins/minerals you'll find your nails will recover nicely.

Mostly I find meats and fish to be very acceptable for most people.

Rice is also good for most people but come off it for 6 months or so if you have a yeast problem. Rice turns into sugar in your body and feeds yeast. *(Soak and wash rice well to remove starch if you suffer with constipation)*

Corn and rye products are generally good. *(Not Sweetcorn)*
*(Don't eat these if you have a **big** yeast problem)*

Wheat suits most people…. Pasta and spaghetti should be okay.
(Come off it for 6 months or so if you have a yeast problem as it turns into sugar in your body and feeds yeast)

If you have noticed little change in your health in the next three months then come off wheat products **SLOWLY** as there is every chance that you have a problem with it in your brain.

Drink **weak** tea/coffee and/or non-carbonated water.

Keep your foods plain and simple where you can.

Try and take a little exercise when you start to feel better and start toning up those muscles again as it all helps you to feel good.

Don't listen to advice from family and friends as I'm sure they mean well but they don't even know what suits their **own** brain much less yours.

Remember this diet is not forever you can go back onto most of the foods in about six to nine months; just feel your way into them slowly. If you feel good then okay, if you don't feel good then come off them again.

FINALLY!…AND THIS IS PROBABLY THE MOST IMPORTANT PIECE OF ADVICE I AM GIVING YOU. IF YOU DO NOT GET YOUR TOOTHPASTE RIGHT THEN YOU HAVE VERY LITTLE OR NO CHANCE OF BEING HEALTHY. *HOMEOPATHIC* IS THE ONLY TOOTHPASTE I HAVE EVER RECOMMENDED BECAUSE IT'S THE MILDEST TOOTHPASTE FOR THE BRAIN TO COPE WITH.

You should find it in most *independent* chemist shops or health food stores. Get 8 or 10 **weak** tasting/smelling flavours and rotate them from day to day. Put only a very small amount on the toothbrush as that's all it takes to clean your teeth. Most of what you would normally fill the brush with goes down the plughole and makes the manufacturer very wealthy. It's the same as mustard on the plate, it's not what's eaten that makes the manufacturer rich but what's thrown away.

Chapter **12**

VITAMINS & MINERALS

A report in the Daily Mail on Monday May 5th 2003 stated that too many vitamins can damage your health. Well, quite frankly I would assume that most of us suspected that already.

The Vitamin and mineral industry is worth some £175 million a year. In this report the UK Food Standards Agency say that the 10 million or so people that buy supplements are effectively wasting their money. They say that a healthy well balanced diet which includes lots of fruit and vegetables will provide all the nutriments that most people need.   My question is **not** about people that have **too many** vitamins and minerals in their body but what about the people that have **too few**?

Vitamins and minerals are the body's essential raw materials. They are the most important things in your body, yet most doctors don't even talk to you about them let alone test to see if you have enough. About **one in five** of the 10,000 people that I've tested for levels of vitamins and minerals actually had a deficiency. You wouldn't drive a car for 20 or 30 years **or more** and not check the oil and water or indeed let them run dry before you put some in. Well vitamins and minerals are your body's oil and water. Your body cannot function correctly if these are deficient. They are the raw materials that are used to make every part of your body, bone skin, teeth etc. They are catalysts for one another so if you are deficient in one then others will not work so effectively. People often say that they get all the vitamins and minerals their body needs from the foods they eat. Well which vitamins and minerals does your body need, is it low on any?

WHY DOCTORS DON'T MAKE YOU HEALTHY.

Has anybody ever checked your levels of vitamins and minerals?

Even if you did know which vitamins and minerals your body needed and you also knew which foods they came in, how many eggs for example would you have to eat per day to get your body's requirement of B12? You have no way of knowing the absorption rate of B12 into your body. The other problem is that with mass production of foods these days the vitamin and mineral content is often quite low, this is due to over farming.

It's common knowledge that there are only so many vitamins and minerals in the soil and these are taken out by the crop but very rarely replaced by the farmer. You only have to look at and taste a home-grown lettuce to appreciate what I am saying here.

Not only will your home-grown lettuce be a darker richer shade of green but it will undoubtedly taste far better than the shop bought one. Another possible problem is that the lettuce itself may well be a harmful drug to your brain and that will lead to other problems of food intolerance if you are eating lots of them in order to get your so-called right amount of vitamins and minerals.

Every doctor you have ever been to should have checked your levels of vitamins and minerals **before** doing anything else, if your levels are low how can you be healthy? There are about 86 known vitamins and minerals in our body but I have not yet found a conventional High Street store selling a combined **'Vitamin and Mineral'** with more than about 40 in it. I have often wondered why they do not sell us **all** the vitamins and minerals our body needs.

Maybe one day somebody from a drug company will explain that one to me.

WHY DOCTORS DON'T MAKE YOU HEALTHY.

My theory is that if they did sell us all the vitamins and minerals that our body needed then we would get healthier and that would be bad for business. Anyway, my advice to you is to go out and buy the combined vitamin and mineral tablets that give you the **most** items in one pill. Count them on the label; don't worry about how many milligrams of each there are just get the one with the most vitamins and minerals in it. Put them into your body on a daily basis and let your body kick out in your urine the ones it doesn't want. Take only the quantity shown on the label and don't leave them in the cupboard or you might as well leave them in the shop. Its cheap insurance so put them into your body every day of your life. Buy only pure vitamins and minerals don't buy them mixed with herbs or any other weird or wonderful things.
I know about Colloidal vitamins and minerals these are in fact very good, they will provide most of the vitamins and minerals the body needs. The problem I find with them though is that they taste very bitter and they often cause stomach upsets. Because they taste a bit weird they're mostly mixed with fruit juice before being sold and fruit juice itself will often cause stomach problems by feeding yeast. So keep it simple and buy standard high street vitamins and minerals in tablet form. If they ever bring out **'Colloidal'** vitamins and minerals in tablet form then go for them and let me know where they are so that I can tell my other patients. For those of you that have never heard of Colloidal vitamins and minerals they are taken directly from the plant rather than from the ground as in conventional high street vitamins and minerals. This makes their particles about a 1,000 times smaller and allows for easier absorption into the body. According to the information I have read over the years the best recorded absorption rate **into** the body of conventional vitamins & minerals was 12.5% and if you look at the colour of your urine after taking them you can see why. Basically the particles are so large they're not going **into** your body but straight **through** it.

Colloidals on the other hand being so small actually absorb into the body very effectively. Another reason that Colloidals are absorbed into the body so well is that they carry a **negative** electrical charge. This is due to the fact that they are taken directly from the plant. Conventional vitamins and minerals are taken from the ground and carry a **positive** electrical charge.

Our body runs on **positive** electrical power so you can see why it rejects conventional vitamins and minerals. It's exactly the same as trying to push two similar magnetic poles together ...you've got no chance.

If you ever get a chance to listen to a CD/tape by: Dr Joel D Wallach (1991 Nobel Prize Nominee-Medicine) then please do, it's entitled: **Dead Doctors Don't Lie!**

It's fantastic, there are some things he says that I don't agree with but I have to admit it makes compulsive listening. He talks about quite a wide range of health matters as well as Colloidals. I'm sure you will find him on the internet; maybe you could order a copy there.

I used to sell my **own label** Colloidal multi-vitamins/minerals years ago. I had them shipped in from the US...but guess what!

A drug company bought my supplier out and closed down the operation. There's a sample Health Scan vitamin and mineral printout shown on page 85. As you will see this patient has a deficiency of Iron and Magnesium.

Caution:
If you are pregnant, diabetic or suffer with a serious disease please consult with your doctor before taking supplements.

Vitamins and minerals tested during a scan are listed below:

1. Calcium
2. Chromium
3. Cobalt
4. Copper
5. Iodine
6. Iron
7. Magnesium
8. Manganese
9. Molybdenum
10. Potassium
11. Selenium
12. Silicon
13. Sodium
14. Zinc
15. Folic Acid (Folacin)
16. Vitamin A (Retinol)
17. Vitamin B1 (Thiamine)
18. Vitamin B2 (Riboflavin)
19. Vitamin B3 (Niacin)
20. Vitamin B5 (Pantothenic Acid)
21. Vitamin B6 (Pyridoxine)
22. Vitamin B12 (Cobalamin)
23. Vitamin C (Ascorbic Acid)
24. Vitamin D (Cholecaciferol)
25. Vitamin E (Tocopherol)
26. Bitumen H (Biotin)
27. Bioflavonoids (Vitamin P Complex)
28. Vitamin K (Coagulation)
29. Boron.

WHY DOCTORS DON'T MAKE YOU HEALTHY.

Item Name	ID	Max ↓	
1. Vitamin B12 (Cobalamin)	001	54	
2. Vitamin C (Ascorbic Acid)	002	54	
3. Cobalt	003	53	
4. Calcium	004	53	
5. Chromium	005	53	
6. Vitamin H (Biotin)	006	53	
7. Bioflavonoids (Vit P Complex)	007	53	
8. Vitamin K (Coagulation)	008	53	
9. Boron	009	53	
10. Vitamin E (Tocopherol)	000	52	**LEVELS**
11. Vitamin B6 (Pyridoxine)	011	52	**CURRENTLY**
12. Vitamin B3 (Niacin)	012	52	**FINE**
13. Vitamin B5 (Pantothenic Acid)	013	52	
14. Vitamin D (Cholecaciferol)	014	52	
15. Vitamin B2 (Riboflavin)	015	51	
16. Vitamin B1 (Thiamin)	016	51	
17. Silicon	017	50	
18. Sodium	018	50	
19. Zinc	019	50	
20. Folic Acid (Folacin)	020	50	
21. Vitamin A (Retinol)	021	50	
22. Manganese	022	50	
23. Molybdenum	023	50	
24. Potassium	024	50	
25. Selenium	025	50	
26. Copper	026	48	
27. Iodine	027	48	
28. Magnesium	028	46	**LEVELS**
29. Iron	029	43	**CURRENTLY LOW**

PART 3

TESTIMONIAL LETTERS

Chapter **13**

DRUGS DON'T CURE YOU THEY JUST MAKE THE DRUG COMPANIES RICH

I get a great deal of satisfaction from making people healthy and its nice when it results in a testimonial letter. Also if you think about it letters are the only way I can prove that what I do actually works, because if people out there have any doubts about the effectiveness of my scanning they can always talk to the people that wrote the letters. Each and every letter is another step forward, another brick **out** of The Establishment wall.

Every letter brings closer the day that this technology will be fully integrated into the world of conventional medicine.

Each and every letter will help to ensure that our children and the children of generations to come will **not** have to suffer unnecessarily at the hands of drug companies and those greedy self-indulgent masters who run our healthcare system. We all know how difficult it is to make time in our busy lives to stop and write a letter but without the evidence of testimonial letters I probably would not now be writing this book. So you and your family would almost certainly have just continued on in the same old way being unhealthy and making drug companies richer.

It would not be realistic to expect everyone to sit down and write a letter of thanks. But the letters I have certainly run into many hundreds and show evidence that my scanning has been responsible for curing a range of more than fifty different health problems. If you ever meet a doctor with such testimonial letters then please do let me have his/her name and contact details as I would very much like to meet them.

Chapter **14**

PAIN

Unless you have injured yourself or worn out a joint which now has two surfaces rubbing together or if a scalpel in an operation has cut through a nerve for example, then there is no physical reason why you should be experiencing pain. Pain is a signal that highlights a **problem** just as a warning light would in your car.

All pain signals come **FROM** your brain!

They **GO** to your joints (*or anywhere else in the body*) but they **COME** from your brain!

Your brain sends out pain signals when you injure yourself or when you put signals in from food/drink or drugs of any kind that it cannot cope with. Try drinking a bottle of Gin and you'll see what I mean. Your brain is no different than any other computer if you put **wrong** signals in then you get **wrong** signals out!
It's your brain's way of saying:

'I don't want that **DRUG!**...(*that signal*) I can't cope with it!'

Pain signals from your brain run down wires called nerves and go to the weakest parts of your body (*i.e. an old injury or worn joint*) as these points have the least resistance. It's the same as water trying to escape from a barrel it will always find the weakest points. Pain can of course also stay in your head where it's called a headache or a migraine.

We will now look at various health problems in some detail.
As we do I shall be quoting from various testimonial letters as well as from comments at lectures I have given to the general public, health groups and doctors around the world.

All original testimonial letters are kept on file.

Chapter 15

ARTHRITIS

I have chosen just a few letters from our vast number of Arthritis testimonials to comment on here.

Mr. W from Richmond Surrey

"An amazing recovery in just six weeks." This gentleman was aged about 30 at the time of the scan and could hardly walk due to the pain. He had been treated for years at a number of hospitals and was making the drug companies very rich by taking handfuls of pills every day. His main intolerance was to Wheat.

Mrs. R from Shropshire

This 25-year-old lady was very sceptical. Well if your own doctor can't cure you how is an Alternative Therapist going to do it? She came because she saw an editorial in the Daily Express written about a little girl whose skin problem I cured. Anyway to cut a long story short her health was in a terrible state, she was suffering with severe muscle and joint pain, digestive problems rashes and breathlessness. She was only five weeks away from her wedding day. She'd been through the mill with conventional medicine, waiting months for appointments and sitting in draughty hospital corridors for hours with dozens of other poor hopefuls. The NHS **'specialists'** had done just about every test under the sun and still they couldn't help her, in fact she was getting worse and all they could offer her were handfuls of pills. Within a week of her scan she started to recover and as she says in her letter she *"felt wonderful on her wedding day."*

Her main problems were Cheese and Fruit. A quote from her letter: *"The doctors kept saying there was nothing wrong with me and tried to suggest that I was a hypochondriac, I am living proof that eating the wrong foods can cause dreadful pain and ill health."*

She sent me a piece of her wedding cake and a photo.

At my request this lady sent a copy of her testimonial letter to the reporter at the Daily Express who had written the original article on the little girl. I had hoped that she would be keen to write a report on this amazing story and other such stories of miraculous recovery due to the work of Health Scan and it's **'drug free'** therapy. I don't know why but I assumed that such an important story could well be of interest to millions of readers of The Daily Express. It seems I was wrong. Curing people as I do is obviously way down their list of priorities because I am still waiting on a call from the newspaper some seven years later.
I don't know about you but if I was a reporter I think I would jump at the chance of the biggest scoop of the century as there are not many stories that I can think of more important than health.

Mr. M from Malaga, Spain
A 69-year-old man who had suffered with severe Rheumatoid Arthritis on and off for most of his life. His main intolerance was to a range of vegetables that he ate regularly.
Quotes from his letter:

"I was so incapacitated I couldn't turn myself over in bed without my wife's assistance."

"I have not had an attack of arthritis since adopting your recommendations."

Mrs. F from Bristol

A 62-year-old lady, she suffered with Arthritis for the past 30 years. It was mainly back and lower body pain; she'd also had a hip replacement. She had been in pain even though she was on a **daily** 100mg dose of anti-inflammatory drugs. *(Another nice little earner for the drug companies)* Within 10 weeks of her scan she had reduced her medication to one tablet every two weeks and guess what!

ALL HER PAIN HAD GONE!

Here's another testimonial letter that was sent to the Daily Express, it's not too late if you guys want to contact me:

intolerance@healthscan.co.uk

Mrs M from Stanmore Middlesex

This lady was officially registered disabled with Chronic Osteo Arthritis. Her main food problems were: Mint and Potatoes. Within a few months she wrote to thank me.

"A thousand thanks for helping me overcome my debilitating condition, the constant arthritic pain has subsided and I feel a different person altogether."

I wonder how many other Chronic Osteo Arthritis **'registered disabled'** people are out there now suffering unnecessarily.

Chapter **16**

ASTHMA

3,400,000 people suffer with Asthma in the UK alone. 1 in 5 of them is a child; it kills 2,000 people every year. That's **40 people a week that die from Asthma** and the best the medical world can offer is a Steroid Inhaler. I've yet to find a case of Asthma that was not helped considerably and/or cured completely following a food intolerance test and elimination of Sugar/Yeast and Mint from the diet. People in Africa and dry dusty deprived countries generally don't suffer with Asthma, it's a **'Western'** health problem. People in deprived countries don't have Sugar/Yeast and Mint....Do they?

In my experience of curing Asthma (*And I do have a lot of experience*) the condition is not **caused** by animals and house dust mite as every allergy specialist will tell you. Whilst these things will certainly aggravate the sensitive nerve endings in the lungs they do not **cause** the problem. The sensitive nerve endings in the lungs are **caused** by food intolerance and/or an intolerance to mint in all its forms...Especially that found in toothpaste.

Okay!...Let's take a look at some Asthma testimonial letters.

Our first letter is from the mum of a beautiful little 4-year old girl. Her parents brought her to see me on the 12th February 2003. Their testimonial letter was written exactly 3 months later on the 12th May 2003. **SHE WAS CURED!**

Here's a bit of background on the case:
She had **severe** Asthma since she was 14 months old.

WHY DOCTORS DON'T MAKE YOU HEALTHY.

She was being treated in England at several specialist hospitals but mostly at The Royal Brompton in South London. In just under three years she made over 50 visits to various hospitals for treatment of her Asthma. She was admitted to intensive care on three of these visits because her condition had become so serious. During her treatment over nearly 3 years the best the NHS could offer her was excessive amounts of Steroids. Within 3 months of her visit to Health Scan she was discharged from hospital and has gone on to enjoy a normal healthy life. Her food test showed a major intolerance to Wheat and Mint! *(Good old toothpaste yet again!)*

In the letter her mum said that the hospital specialists acknowledged that she was cured but refused to accept that her recovery was food related. Just how blatantly ignorant and stubborn can any doctor be to refuse to accept such overwhelming evidence, they see it with their own eyes yet they **still** refuse to accept it. This applies not just in this case but also in the many thousands of other cases of people I've cured over the years. The doctors all preferred to keep their heads in the sand rather than openly accept that their patients had been cured by an Alternative Therapist. So with that in mind is it not reasonable for the remaining patients of these doctors to question as to **why** they to are not being notified of this particular treatment. Surely the patients should be given the right to make up their own minds and to choose which treatment they prefer. If there is a cure out there and these doctors are aware of it then why do they allow their patients to continue to suffer unnecessarily?

NHS doctors are public employees and as such they should be ethically, morally and legally bound to divulge such information to us their employer. Also, if a doctor is aware that treatment such as food intolerance testing can and does cure these major health problems then why can we **the public** not take legal action against a doctor for not divulging it? In the case of each and every one of the thousands of patients that I've cured their GP or hospital specialist should at least have enquired as to **how** this was achieved. You can count on one hand the number of doctors that have done so. Is it not unreasonable therefore to judge that the doctors in question had their **own interests** at heart rather than that of their patients?

Or could there be some financial reason? Surely not!

Mind you, if there was what a case there would be to answer.

There must be some reason for it though.

Mrs L from Surrey

"Since she has been tested her life is one that we could only have dreamed of."

That quote is from the letter of a mum of an 8-year-old girl.

She had been in and out of hospital all her life suffering with Asthma excessive coughing and weight loss. The doctors prescribed steroid inhalers and various other medications.

Within four months of her Health Scan she was discharged from hospital and made a full recovery. But just look at the foods that were causing her health problems, good **'balanced diet type foods'** such as Cows milk!…Potatoes!…Vegetables!…Sugar! and wait for it!...Yes…Good old **mint** toothpaste!

You would think also that the hospital specialists treating this girl for **eight years** would have shown **some** interest in how she was cured and by whom. It's now five years later and I'm still waiting for him/her/them to contact me but as I said previously it's the same with virtually **'ALL'** doctors of patients I've cured with the exception of one or two. The only time I hear from doctors is when they themselves want treatment. You'd be amazed at the amount of doctors/dentists/nutritionists and other so-called health professionals both conventional and complimentary that I've treated and cured over the years.

WHY DOCTORS DON'T MAKE YOU HEALTHY.

Father M from London
"I thank god for the day I went to Health Scan."
Hey!…That's not bad considering it was written by a Catholic priest!…At least I'm in with the right people, there's hope for me and this technology yet!

This gentleman had a huge yeast problem that was being made worse by his altar wine.

He'd have been waiting a long time for his doctor to find that one!

He suffered severe breathing problems from time to time that brought on panic attacks and so it was a vicious circle of pills and sprays and more pills and sprays.
(No complaints from the drug companies though!)

Mrs M from Kingston Surrey
A middle-aged lady, she suffered with Asthma for **20 years.**
Her cure took 6 weeks.

"From the age of 22 I have suffered with Asthma and since visiting your clinic six weeks ago I have not had to use my inhaler once. I am so pleased that my Asthma is now a thing of the past and I cannot recommend Health Scan enough."

Mrs T from Abu Dhabi
This letter is from the mum of an Arab boy aged 10 who had suffered the whole of his life with severe Asthma.

He was cured within 3 weeks of his scan!

What was he intolerant to?
Yeast!…And yes, you've guessed it, our old favourite mint!

"I'm writing to thank you for what you have done for my son, you were our last hope. No more medicines or inhalers…you don't know what a relief that is. He was cured within 3 weeks of his scan and he's been free from Asthma now for two months, he feels and looks great."

CLEAN HOMES ARE ASTHMA RISK

That was a headline in The Daily Mail of December 23rd 2004.
"The cleaner you're home the more likely it is that your child will develop Asthma… say medical researchers." The report was written by a doctor and blamed household sprays for the 100% increase in Asthma over the past 10 years. These findings were based on the fact that sales of such products have increased by 60% during that time. I do hope this research was not funded by public money for if it wasn't so serious such findings could be considered a joke. The facts of this no doubt costly **'medical'** research would have been better published on the 1st of April.

Eczema has also increased considerably over the past 10 years but that's probably due to the fact that there has been a 150% increase in the sale of wallpaper. Now maybe I can get a **huge** government grant to support my vital research for the next 5 years.

Chapter 17

CELIAC DISEASE

Celiac Disease is the inability to tolerate Gluten and Wheat protein.

The symptoms are:

> Abdominal distension
> Vomiting
> Diarrhoea
> Lethargy
> Foul smelling stools

But guess what.

It's not a disease…. It's a yeast problem!

I've cured vast numbers of patients who were misdiagnosed with Celiac disease.

(I wonder how much taxpayer's money is spent each year on research into Celiac disease.)

Chapter **18**

CHRONIC FATIGUE SYNDROME (M.E.)

The medical name of this condition is:
MYALGIC ENCEPHALOMYELITIS

Basically it's a condition that doctors know **'nothing'** about.

Skytext: Sunday March 4th 2004
Hundreds of M.E. sufferers demonstrated outside parliament to demand better research into M.E.
It costs the British taxpayer £3.5 billion p.a.
There are 240,000 registered sufferers in the UK, some are as young as 5.
Action for M.E. (Charity) has called for more research.

Hello there!…Is there anybody listening at Action M.E?

This condition is caused by food intolerance!

There are many symptoms but the main ones could well be considered to be severe lack of energy and muscular weakness.
More often than not people are diagnosed with M.E. when doctors have tried and failed with routine medication.
The patients are mostly told there's nothing wrong with them and all that's needed is for them to pull themselves together.

What an insult!
M.E. is Food Intolerance **EVERY** time! How do I know?
Well I've cured all the M.E. sufferers that I've treated.

WHY DOCTORS DON'T MAKE YOU HEALTHY.

I was watching the B.B.C. TV Breakfast show on the morning of December 17th 2002. It featured reports on M.E. and various cases of the condition that the medical profession was struggling to treat. Patients were complaining of the lack of help they received so I immediately emailed the show and attached a P.R. report on how my scanning works.

Here's my email:

From: GERARD KIELTY I.R.B; I.D.E.
To: Breakfastplanning@bbc.co.uk
Sent: 17 December 2002 12:00
Subject: HEALTH SCAN (Re: M.E.)

Hello and Good Morning,

Having tuned into your programme at 8:30 this morning I heard you talking about M.E. I am an Alternative Health Practitioner specialising in the field of Food Intolerance. I have treated many hundreds if not thousands of M.E. sufferers successfully over the last 10 years. It is a condition that the medical profession diagnose when they have no idea just what is wrong with you.
I have yet to find a case of M.E. that I have not cured completely with a **SINGLE** Food Intolerance test. Patients become healthy within six weeks on average and **NO** drugs are required.
Please do take a look at the attached press release as this will explain in detail just how my scanning works. My website is currently down as it's having work done on it but if you decide to investigate this item further then I will get them to switch it back on so that you can access the vast amount of info therein. I have cured about 10,000 people over the last 10 years **WITHOUT** drugs and I treat a range of some 50 different health problems.

However, if you would like to work with me and advertise for say 50 people suffering with M.E. and if you are prepared to film my work then I will come to your studio and scan them all for free and **'cure'** them all within about 2 months.

Unfortunately drug companies and doctors in general have a vested interest in not advancing this technology as it cures people without drugs. So can I suggest that if we are to proceed then let it be on the basis that we do it on our own. Do not look for guidance from your resident/staff G.P. or medical advisers.
This technology can and will become the future of healthcare when enough people know of it and what it can do. Between us we can get the message to the masses and then the politicians and medical professionals will have to come up with a convincing answer as to why they do not allow the public to have such treatment when it cures so many health problems so simply and without the need for drugs of any kind. From a business point of view drug companies should not be interested in curing people as they make no money from healthy people!

Governments are always complaining about the cost of health treatment (especially the NHS) this technology would release billions of £'s each and every year that could be put to better use and most of all it will cure generations to come without the need for drugs. This is the future of medicine! This in effect could well be the most important news story of the century and all it would take is about 3 months to put it together. If you want to work with me then I will be happy to send on a vast amount of P.R. material as well as recordings of Radio & TV interviews that I have done over the years. To date such interviews have been on small local TV & Radio so their impact has been restricted.

If I can have a chance to show the world my work on the B.B.C. then we will change global healthcare systems forever.

I will leave you with the fact that in my work of curing some 10,000 people I have found **VEGETABLES** are a major cause of health problems. **Yes VEGETABLES!**
I know it's hard to believe but it's true.
HEROIN is a drug that grows in the ground. Well a lettuce also grows in the ground so why is this not a drug too?
It is a drug!
And if you think that's weird then let me tell you that the biggest cause of health problems, way out in front of all others is
MINT TOOTHPASTE!
About 95% of the 10,000 people I've tested were intolerant to it.

And who makes toothpaste?

DRUG COMPANIES!

Please email me a.s.a.p.   intolerance@healthscan.co.uk
I look forward to your reply.

 GERARD KIELTY I.R.B; I.D.E.

www.healthscan.co.uk

That email was sent on the 17th December 2002 and a reply was further requested on the 2nd January 2003.
It's now March 2006…nothing yet!
Obviously they're not interested but the least they should have done was to reply or am I just being unreasonable again?

B.B.C. salaries are paid by the taxpayer via the TV licence. So just as with doctors it could be argued that B.B.C. staff have a moral obligation to their employers (**the public**) to ensure that they inform them of such a breakthrough in healthcare technology. If you could find a human to talk to at the BBC (rather than a computerised switchboard that sends you round in ever decreasing circles) then I am sure they would claim in their defence that they get thousands of emails every day. Yes!…I'm sure they do but why have a system that takes viewers emails if you are not prepared to reply to them. Or do they get thousands of emails every day from people claiming to be able to **cure** over 50 different health problems without drugs?

There are literally millions of people out there watching their TV channel every day that could live a life free of health problems if the powers that be at the BBC chose to inform them.

Maybe someone from the BBC will now contact me with a view to following up my letter. It's never too late you know but I won't hold my breath.

You can get me at…intolerance@healthscan.co.uk

I presume that emails like mine just get **deleted** by doctors that are employed by the BBC to sort and answer incoming medical enquiries.

Note: I also emailed Action for M.E. on the 17th December 2002 and yes you've guessed it!…I'm still awaiting their reply also.

I have received a great many testimonials from M.E sufferers that I've treated but I will now quote from just two.

Mrs C from Scotland

This 50-year-old lady had trouble walking up four steps into my clinic, 3 months later she was climbing mountains in Scotland.

"After 5 years of severe ME I am writing to thank you for giving me back my life. I am just back from a holiday in the Lake District where I managed to climb two fells one at 1500 and the

other at 2500 feet. People are asking me about the test espec...
when they see how well I look after 5 years of really poor health.

Miss H from Richmond Surrey

A young lady of 24 she was put on anti-depressants by her specialist and told to give up looking for a job.

What great advice for a 24 year old!

Three months after coming to Health Scan she was cured.

"After four years of constant fatigue, repeated illness and violent mood swings I was diagnosed as having ME. I was advised to take anti-depressants and to give up looking for a job (I had just finished my degree). Three months after my scan I feel better than I have for years. I no longer get up in the morning panicking about the fact that it will be another 10 hours before I can sleep again. I now feel like a healthy 24 year old instead of an unhealthy 80 year old."

Chapter **19**

ONCENTRATION

When you do **not** poison your brain your health problems will go away and you can also look forward to a **vast** increase in concentration. You'll find it's amazing just how well your brain **can and will** run your body when you **stop** poisoning it.

Remember!…it's your **brain** that runs your body and **not** your **taste buds** or **stomach**. Nothing happens in your body that is not controlled **by** your brain. *(Apart from the fermentation of yeast)*

As in the case of the 13-year-old lad with Hay Fever who's schoolwork improved so dramatically (see Hay Fever section) we see yet again how food intolerance effects everything in our body **including** our concentration and memory. Just as in this lad's case its **not** that we've forgotten something; the problem is that because our brain is being poisoned with **bad** drugs it isn't able to concentrate and **absorb** information in the first place. So if the information is not taken **in** by the brain then how can it be there to be recalled at a later date? We have all been introduced to a stranger only to find that 5 minutes later we can't remember their name. It's not that we couldn't **remember** their name, the problem is that we didn't **hear it** in the first place! We were not concentrating when we were introduced and the name went straight **over** our heads instead of going **into** our brain.

With regard to increased concentration…*(and energy levels)* whilst I obviously can't mention names I can tell you that I've scanned a number of top football teams in the (UK) Premier League. And that's one of the main reasons **why they are** top teams! Once they've been scanned each and every player is finely tuned to their **own** brain requirements and as a result of not being poisoned their brain wakes up fully. Their energy and concentration levels increase dramatically and they are then one step ahead of the opposition. Although they play in a team sport each and every player is an individual, they all have their own unique brain so there's no point in treating them all the same when it comes to diet.

In addition to those above I've scanned many top sports people such as:

GOLFERS - RUGBY PLAYERS - SNOOKER PLAYERS

TENNIS PLAYERS - SWIMMERS - ATHLETES

also JOCKEYS and their HORSES.

Yes!...I've even scanned racehorses!
The results have been amazing!
When you think about it horses have a brain and a nervous system so why shouldn't they suffer from food intolerance?

They do!

If we as humans can get Migraine/Arthritis or any other health problem from food intolerance then why can't a horse or any other animal? They won't run very well with a migraine will they!

Chapter **20**

CROHN'S DISEASE

This disease causes inflammation of the bowel.

The symptoms are:

> Nausea
>
> Lethargy
>
> Weight loss
>
> Diarrhoea
>
> Abdominal pain
>
> Weakness.

It's another yeast problem!

I've cured an awful lot of people over the years that were diagnosed with Crohn's Disease when I treated them for yeast.

Did you know that £250 million of taxpayer's money is spent each and every year on NHS treatment of Crohn's Disease?

It's a crazy world!

No wonder they can't afford to pay the nurses, paramedics and other non-management staff a decent living wage.

And finally, as if there wasn't enough problems out there already with sugar a chocolate manufacture announced a scheme in 2003 to give **FREE** basketball nets to schools if and when children sent in **X** amount of chocolate bar wrappers.

Did you know that there's **£4 BILLION** worth of chocolate eaten in the UK each year. (Info source: B.B.C. news 29/4/03)

Chapter **21**

ECZEMA / DERMATITIS

According to the BBC website there are 6 million people suffering with eczema in the UK. If there are 6 million sufferers in the UK then god knows how many there are throughout the world. The crazy thing is that I have yet to find a skin problem that I've not cured with a **'SINGLE'** food intolerance test. I wonder how many hundreds of so-called NHS specialist hospitals and clinics there are out there living off us the taxpayer and off Drug Company funding while pretending to cure their patients?

General advice:

You'll find that your skin problems will slowly clear as you come off the problem foods but in the meantime it's a good idea to lubricate your skin. I recommend that you use only Aloe Vera skin cream *(get it as pure as possible)*. Patch test a little on the back of your leg for 12 hours or so before using it elsewhere on your body. I've always recommended Aloe Vera for the first few weeks of treatment of skin problems *(do not drink it)* it's a product that generally does a good job and it seems to suit most people but stop using it once your skin has healed. For those of you with excessive skin problems you would be wise to pop into your local chemist and ask for an antiseptic *(plastic)* skin spray. If you spray the area affected this will seal the damage within seconds and help to speed up the healing time.

Tip: Keep a bottle of Aloe Vera in the kitchen as it's great for immediate treatment of minor burns. More serious burns should be treated with **'running'** cold water until medical help arrives.

Our first letter is from a 21-year-old lady who had tried every conceivable remedy. She like most eczema sufferers had of course seen numerous NHS specialists and been prescribed vast quantities of that old favourite **STEROID** cream. I'm sure I don't have to tell any of you the problems that wonderful stuff causes.

Miss P from London

*"I have suffered from eczema since childhood and at the age of 21 I thought I'd tried every available remedy, Chinese herbs, acupressure, various creams and bandages, Dead Sea mineral baths...the list is endless. After years of NHS prescribed steroid creams my skin had become thin and even more sensitive, I looked and felt a mess. So I had a Health Scan and now just a few months later I feel **GOOD!** My skin has cleared and it's now smooth and itchless, fellow eczema sufferers will understand my joy. I believe this test should be made compulsory for all as it's a turning point in my life and is the best thing I've ever done."*

Our second letter is from a very nice lady that suffered with itchy skin for a great many years. On scratching she would make her skin bleed and of course this would just inflame the condition.

Mrs S from Marbella

"I have had very bad and itchy skin on my arms and back for years. My scan showed that I was intolerant to Olive Oil which amazed me as I had always thought it to be healthy. I cooked with it rubbed it onto my skin and even made soap from it. It has only been a few months since my scan but my skin is now smooth and it doesn't itch anymore."

Note how Olive Oil was such a disaster for this lady. It is typical of how marketing works for if you tell people enough times that something is **good for them** or that its **healthy** then eventually they will start to believe it.

WHY DOCTORS DON'T MAKE YOU HEALTHY.

Miss J from Middlesex

*"This service was recommended to me by a work colleague who had earlier benefited from your test. He assured me that your scanning would identify the cause of my skin disorders such as continuous rashes and inflammation. To my amazement after one month it had made such an incredible difference to my complexion, it was like one of those '**before**' and '**after**' health service adverts and it actually worked. I am very grateful for the service you offer and appreciate the manner in which it's explained and carried out. I would recommend Health Scan to everyone."*

I have treated many hundreds of people with **severe** skin problems but this young man has to be the worst of all.

Mr M from Nottingham

"Ever had an annoying itch? ...I had one! ...When I scratched it my skin would start weeping and wouldn't stop, most of my body was in this condition including my face. I looked and felt like something from a horror show. My doctor prescribed antihistamines, sensitive skin moisturiser and hydrocortisone. These were having limited success and I felt uneasy about the side effects. Liver function tests showed that I would need a new liver if I continued with the antihistamines and I know that hydrocortisone discolours the skin with prolonged use. One day my friend's mother read a whole page article in the Daily Express about a child with skin problems that had been cured by Health Scan. I booked an appointment and within weeks I attended their clinic feeling drained, sceptical, embarrassed and desperate. I was met by friendly reception staff that were pleasant despite my very unpleasant appearance.

I know that sometimes we are told that things will not hurt just to give us confidence. In this case I was surprised because there was absolutely no pain it was just like touching the end of your finger with a ball point pen. I left the clinic and felt that I had just been given some big answers and now had hope of a cure.

WITHIN TWO WEEKS MY SKIN HAD HEALED!

After 6 months I had another Liver function test and it showed that all was normal again."

A copy of this letter was also sent to a reporter at The Daily Express.

Won't be long now!

The child referred to above in the Daily Express whole page article is called Holly, her mother wrote to me on Tuesday February 20th 1996. Holly was six then and she'd been suffering with severe eczema most of her life. Her biggest problem turned out to be Olive Oil and mum had been rubbing this into her skin trying to lubricate the dry sore and very itchy condition.
Holly used to cry herself to sleep each night whilst in pain from scratching. Holly had been under numerous hospital specialists and dieticians for years. Holly was cured within **TWO** weeks of her visit to Health Scan. What I don't understand is how the reporter from the Express newspaper could receive yet another testimonial letter telling of incredible success with health problems and not follow it up as anybody with journalistic instincts surely would. I know that Health Scan is not the only story in the world and I'm sure that reporters have many other things to do each day but just stop for a moment and consider yourself in their shoes. You're a freelance journalist and you write an article about food intolerance and it's published by a national newspaper, okay great you make some money, end of story. But hold on a moment letters keep coming in from people telling you how they have been cured after a lifetime of suffering

following a single food intolerance test. I don't know about you but as a journalist I'd think that I'd struck gold and be hot on the trail of the story. Can you imagine you have just stumbled across probably the biggest story ever and with a bit of research from the patients involved you would have thousands of health reports that every newspaper and magazine throughout the world would snap up. Anyway for those of you at the Express or any other publication my email address is still: intolerance@healthscan.co.uk

Mrs N from Norway
This lady had been treated by conventional medicine for 15 years both at her home in Norway and at several other hospitals and clinics throughout the world. When she returned to show her local dermatologist the great results he just shrugged his shoulders and walked off. You would think as a so-called **caring** health professional that he might at least have asked to speak with me. This lady had major intolerance to Wheat several vegetables and to Cod Liver Oil, which of course she had been taking on a daily basis for years. The following photographs were taken some five months after she visited my clinic but her skin had healed within a few months of her scan.

I will say no more as the photographs speak for themselves.

(These can be seen in colour on my website)

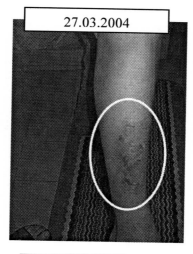

27.03.2004

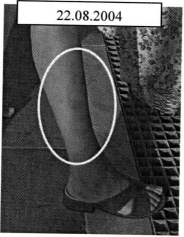

22.08.2004

Figure 7. Rash on leg before and after.

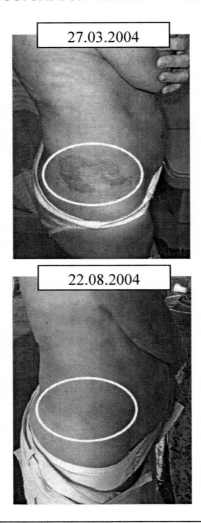

Figure 8: Rash on Torso; before and after.

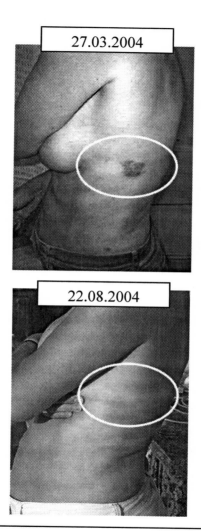

Figure 9: Rash on upper Torso; before and after.

Chapter 22

EPILEPSY

There are an estimated 400,000 epileptics in the UK and 1 in 4 of them are children. If you look in any medical dictionary it tells you that epilepsy is caused by '*interference to the normal electrical function of the brain.*' Well, if you eat an apple and your brain is **intolerant** to the signal **from** that apple then that to is **going to interfere** with the **normal** electrical function of the brain. Not so many years ago they used to lock people away in mental institutions if they suffered with epilepsy. In fact the brother of one of our best known UK film actors (whom I've scanned) was one such case, he spent 70 years of his life behind bars with all sorts of crazy and dangerous people. One treatment for epilepsy still being used today in the NHS is Electro Convulsive Therapy and in my opinion it's just as barbaric as any medieval torture. They actually strap patients to a chair and give them a **major** electric shock to the head/brain!...**Yes!**...**That's real 21st century medicine that is!** If you ask me it's the doctors that do it that should be strapped to the chair. How can they even begin to call themselves doctors when they do such things to other human beings? **God!...it's like Nazi Germany!** The electric shocks more often than not cause convulsions so it's a vicious circle and the poor patients *(victims)* are in a no win situation.

In my work as a paramedic I visited many mental hospitals with patients. I will now try and describe the scene and mood of such a place as most of you reading this will fortunately have no such knowledge of these establishments. When reading try and imagine yourself being sent there as a child suffering with epilepsy as has happened many thousands of times.

For the purpose of this short scene I am taking a *(non-patient)* lady by the name of Paula for her first visit to a mental hospital.

SETTING THE SCENE:
AS WE ENTER THE MAIN GATES THE LOUD CRACKLE OF CAR TYRES ON LOOSE GRAVEL CAN BE HEARD.
I DRIVE SLOWLY UP THE LONG AND TWISTING DRIVEWAY AS A HUGE VICTORIAN 'CREEPY' RED BRICKED BUILDING COMES INTO VIEW.
ABANDONED OVERGROWN HEDGES LINE THE ROUTE.
ON THE GRASS OFF TO OUR RIGHT THERE'S A HALF BROKEN AND ANCIENT LOOKING SIGN WITH THE BARELY READABLE WORDS:

* NO HOPE MENTAL HOSPITAL *

"My God!... says Paula*...it's like something out of a Dracula movie!"*

I know!…It gives me the creeps every time I come here, imagine having to live here. Even worse imagine having to live here as a child! There's an awful lot of places like this around the country that they hide people away in and they **never ever** see the light of day again."

"My God!" …says Paula in a low frightened whisper.

WE STOP THE CAR BY THE 'HUGE' FRONT DOOR OF THE BUILDING AND WALK CAUTIOUSLY ON THE NOISY STONES. THERE'S NOT A SOLE TO BE SEEN.

I OPEN THE CREAKING DIRTY (UNPAINTED) FRONT DOOR AND WE WALK INTO A LONG DARK EYRIE CORRIDOR. DISTANT NOISES SUCH AS CHANTING AND COUGHING CAN BE HEARD. WE HEAR WHAT SOUNDS LIKE HEAVY DOORS SLAMMING IN THE DISTANCE. THE WALLS AND FLOORS ARE COVERED IN DARK (MOULDY) GREEN TILES FOR AS FAR AS THE EYE CAN SEE. ALTHOUGH IT'S STILL DAY TIME THE LIGHTS ARE ON SO AS TO ILLUMINATE THIS ALMOST WINDOWLESS CORRIDOR. THERE'S A STALE SMELL OF EXCREMENT AND BODY SWEAT IN THE AIR AND A SMOKY HAZE THAT BURNS THE EYES.

A COUPLE OF MALE NURSES DRESSED IN DIRTY WHITE UNIFORMS WALK TOWARDS US.
ONE OF THEM IS SWINGING A HUGE CHAINED KEYRING WITH LOTS OF KEYS ON IT.

THEY PASS WHILST TALKING WITHOUT THE SLIGHTEST INDICATION THAT THEY'VE SEEN US. THERE ARE 5 OR 6 PATIENTS MOVING ABOUT IN THE CORRIDOR WEARING 'SCRUFFY' PIN STRIPED PYJAMAS AND SLIPPERS. SOME ARE WALKING VERY CLOSE BEHIND OTHERS WHILST A FEW CHANT WEIRD UNRECOGNISABLE SOUNDS. THEY 'ALL' LOOK AS THOUGH THEY'VE NOT BEEN WASHED IN YEARS. THEY WALK IN A SLOW HEAD DOWN FASHION AS THEY STAY CLOSE TO THE WALLS

"God!...Says Paula in a low shocked whisper... *It's like something from another world!...The poor devils!..I had no idea this sort of thing even existed!*"

WHY DOCTORS DON'T MAKE YOU HEALTHY.

You ain't seen nothing yet! This is the good stuff! These are the lucky ones! Most of them in here have never even **seen** the corridor, much less **walked** in it!

"Oh! My God," replies Paula in shock and disbelief.

Imagine being locked in here all your life Paula because you suffer with epilepsy or depression when both conditions are easily curable with a single food intolerance test. The medical world should be ashamed. It has a great deal to answer for.

.....................The End.....................

I cured an epileptic child in Abu Dhabi UAE with a **single** food intolerance test. His doctors *(the best that money could buy)* said he was incurable as he had too much electricity in the left side of his brain. Wow! If these are the **best** doctors then it doesn't say much for the rest of them.

A lady aged about 25 came to see me with Status Epilepticus she had been having anything up to **20 fits a day** since she was 5 years old and she'd been pumped full of medication throughout those 20 years. Within 4 months of her scan she had only **2 minor fits** in total. Her hospital professor had to accept that I'd cured her but he refused to see her again if she mentioned Health Scan or came near my clinic.
Yes!... A real caring and professional approach that is!

Dr Andrew Haulton a senior consultant at Leicester Royal Infirmary has been found guilty by the G.M.C. of misdiagnosing and treating Epilepsy. Apparently he gave some 600 patients *(mostly children)* drugs for Epilepsy when in fact they did not have the condition. In a great many of these cases the children suffered severe side effects from these drugs. One would have expected the G.M.C. to have struck Dr Haulton off the medical register for such blatant and dangerous practice over a great many years.   But **NO!**...Our great protector the G.M.C. have allowed him to continue to practice and only placed **restrictions** on his work for the next three years.

Chapter **23**

GOUT

I know that doctors think gout is linked to over production of uric acid in the body but they are wrong. Gout is muscle cramp! It really is as simple as that. Your brain runs your muscles so stop poisoning your brain and your gout will disappear. God knows how many people suffer unnecessarily with this very painful condition. Over the years I have received many letters that refer to gout being cured at Health Scan but one letter in particular is worth a mention. This gentleman suffered so badly with gout that he could hardly walk. He was so very close to selling his electrical business as he could no longer cope. A life on **invalid benefit** was all he had to look forward to. He was another failed case at his local NHS hospital.

Mr P from Surrey

*"After **years** of NHS treatment and **scores** of useless drugs I am delighted to tell you that your testing has totally cleared up my very painful gout. I will never take food for granted again. I will of course recommend your service to everyone and I wish you continued success with your incredible computerised solution."*

How do these doctors continue to justify their existence? If they actually cured people one wouldn't mind but that is very seldom the case. If you or I ran a business that was as unsuccessful as the NHS we would never have got it off the ground in the first place. But who's counting? It's only public money; it's there to be used by those who control it. If NHS management was held personally responsible for spending our money wisely then just as in any other business they would question why funds are being squandered and abused in such a way and to such an alarming degree.

Note: Do avoid **Tonic Water** as it's a major cause of Gout.

Chapter **24**

HAY FEVER / RHINITIS

These two conditions are basically the same thing, which is:

*Inflammation of the mucus membrane of the nose
and sometimes increased eye sensitivity*

But why do the mucus membranes and eyes become inflamed and sensitive? For the very simple reason that your brain has sent wrong signals down wires called nerves **to** your eyes and mucus membranes. And the reason your brain has sent out these wrong signals is due to the fact that you've put wrong signals in.

Doctors will tell you that pollens/grass/dusts/animals etc are the cause of Hay Fever and Rhinitis.

WRONG!

Those items don't **cause** the condition they just **aggravate** it.

How do I know?...*I hear you ask*

Well I've cured all the people that came to me with Hay fever and Rhinitis. As I've just said the above items only aggravate the sensitive nerve endings in the nose and eyes and make the condition worse, they don't actually **cause** the condition in the first place. According to the BBC website there are some nine million Hay Fever suffers in the UK. I wonder how many there are in the world? Most people with Hay Fever and Rhinitis end up sitting in hospital corridors for countless hours waiting for allergy tests to be carried out. Allergy testing is **not** the solution to these conditions.

It might interest you to look at a doctor's report which was printed in The Daily Express of May 30th 2000.

Report:
Only **five** NHS clinics have full time allergy specialists, even with both full and part time staff there is only **1** specialist for every **2.1 million** people in Great Britain. There is currently a 2 year waiting list for allergy testing. The report shows how one patient was monitored over a number of years of NHS treatment and it shows the cost of her treatment as an in-patient at £40,000 and as an outpatient at £27,000.

Some service eh!

I don't know about you but I had to look **twice** at the cost of her treatment, those figures are just unbelievable and this is just for **one** patient! It's no wonder the NHS is in such a mess; what a complete and utter waste of taxpayers money. I'd be interested to hear how both the Minister for Health and our wonderful Hospital Management justify such gross incompetence.

Outpatient costs for this patient were £27,000.

God all mighty!...What did they do for her?

Did they lay on a chauffeur driven Rolls Royce to and from all the hospitals she visited? Did they put her up overnight in 5 star hotels when she came for her appointments? How can the NHS justify spending £27,000 on treating an outpatient?

And if you think that's bad then just take a look at the cost of treating an allergy patient in hospital.... **£40,000!!!**

Multiply those figures by the number of patients being treated in hospitals and I don't just mean for allergies but for any one of the 53 or more different health problems that I cure with a **single** food intolerance test and you will see where your taxes are going. Can you even begin to imagine the savings that would be made if every NHS patient were tested for food intolerance? I'll leave you to do the sums on that one but make sure your sitting down when you press the = button. The above report was written by a Dr Hammond and I must say I like her closing words: *"My guess is that after a bit of reading and a few phone calls you'll know more about allergies than your GP."* I can tell you for sure that after a bit of reading *(especially this book)* you **will** know more about **food intolerance** than your GP.

Okay!...Let's have a look at some Hay Fever/Rhinitis letters.

Our first letter is from the mum of a 13-year-old boy.
The poor lad suffered for many years with severe hay fever but a single visit to Health Scan cured him. His schoolwork also improved as his brain was no longer being sent wrong drugs *(taken as food)* it actually worked properly for the first time and his marks virtually doubled in all the main subjects.

Mrs C from Middlesex
"My son is so much better and his whole life has changed. He used to have lots of days off school with swollen itchy eyes blocked nose and lack of sleep due to his condition. Now he is healthy and enjoying life to the full. His schoolwork has even taken his teachers by surprise for he came top in German and nearly top in English and Maths. These were all subjects that he had previously been struggling with."

The next letter will once again show how much time and *(taxpayer's)* money is being wasted day after day in our wonderful NHS hospitals as this lady spent years trouping around numerous hospitals and undergoing a vast array of useless tests.
To add insult to injury her so-called specialists were making matters worse by pumping her full of antibiotics. *(Yeast!)*

Miss K from Essex
"It all began in 1988 with terrible headaches, constant catarrh and runny nose. I visited my GP nearly three times a month and received antibiotics about every twelve weeks when the sinus pain became unbearable. I spent many long hours in various hospitals undergoing tests for numerous things but nothing was found. As I lived in the countryside my GP felt that my condition might improve if I moved to the city. So I took her advice and moved house only to find that my condition got considerably worse. Since my scan I am feeling fantastic. I can't thank you enough keep up the good work."

Can you believe it, the most advanced medical equipment and brains in the world and the best they could come up with was to tell her to move house...**Incredible!** So in desperation she took her GP's advice and moved house only to find that it made her condition worse.

Surprise!...Surprise!

Never mind...the good news is that her GP doesn't have to bother with her anymore; she's got rid of her at last. I'd imagine that this young lady would have a good case against her GP to claim for **all** expenses incurred in moving house and to claim damages for the disruption to her life as a result of following such pathetic unprofessional and downright useless advice.

And the same compensation rights should apply to all patients that are messed about and often made worse by our great healthcare professionals. Where a patient's **health** and **life** has been totally devastated by incompetent doctors and a simple test *(i.e. food intolerance)* is subsequently found to cure that patient and when the medical world continuously ignores such testing then surely that patient should be at liberty to sue for damages.

Our next letter is a real NHS clanger!
This patient suffered 15 years of **unsuccessful** NHS treatment. This waste of many thousands of pounds of taxpayer's money included two failed nasal operations.

Mrs W from Wiltshire
"Since my visit to you some three months ago my nasal problems have cleared up. After fifteen years of breathing difficulties and endless hospital visits it's such a relief to be able to breathe properly again. I am delighted also to see that your service is advertised at Kingston Hospital where I had my first unsuccessful nasal operation."

One of her two operations was carried out at Kingston Hospital in Surrey; my clinic was only a few miles from that hospital. At the time of treating and **curing** this patient I was advertising my scanning service at several locations **inside** Kingston Hospital. The company that handled such advertising approached me and I thought it would be a first class place to promote my work. After about a week of display I received a letter from the hospital management telling me that my advertising had been removed and they gave no reason why they had taken this action. Needless to say I had great pleasure in sending them a copy of the above letter.

But it was strange!…They didn't reply.

Chapter **25**

HYPERACTIVITY

I've scanned a great many hyperactive children over the years and in just about every case they have made a full recovery. If you think about it some people drink a bottle of whisky and become very hyperactive, they may want to fight with you or just jump around and do silly things. Quite simply what they have done is to poison their brain and as a result their brain sends out weird signals. Well if you poison your brain with **food** it will also send out weird signals. In my opinion all hyperactive children should be tested for food intolerance **before** any medication is prescribed.

As you may know the correct term for this condition is: **Attention Deficit Hyperactivity Disorder...(ADHD)**...But did you know that it's considered by the medical world to be a:

Mental illness!

Let us now look in detail at an interesting article which was published in The Sunday Express of the 9th September 2001 it looks at a report published by:

The Journal of the American Medical Association

This article states that over **20,000** hyperactive children in Britain are being prescribed the drug **Ritalin** and that some of these children are as young as two years of age. It goes on to say that schools have refused to teach hyperactive children unless they are on this drug. It also says that school managers actively promote the use of **Ritalin** and that they get a hefty grant from the government for every child that's on it.

But listen to this:

Ritalin is reported to be more addictive than **Cocaine** and its side-effects are: **Hallucinations, Suicidal Tendencies Derangement** and a **Zombie** like state. The report also says that long term use may cause brain damage. There's also another report in The Sunday Express of November 4th 2001 that links **Ritalin** to **Cancer**. It's frightening isn't it? We live in one of the most medically advanced countries in the world and yet the best we can offer these poor unfortunate kids is to risk giving them Cancer and turning them into Zombies. I have received a vast number of testimonial letters from grateful parents on this condition but I have picked just one to highlight here. It's from a boy of 12 that I scanned and it's a very special letter because he wrote it himself. It's difficult enough to encourage adults to find the time to stop and write letters but when I get one from a child that I've cured then that's very special indeed.

Thank you Paul.

Paul from Cleethorpes

"I am writing to say that the test you did is working very well.
It's helped in lots of different ways in my life like at school with maths, English, science, reading etc. My behaviour is much better and I can now restrain myself a lot more than I ever could before. All my grades have gone up and I am more popular with the kids and teachers at my school. It was hard being different to all the kids at school and at home and being shouted at by my parents and teachers. My life is a lot easier now so I am writing to say a big THANK YOU."

Chapter **26**

IRRITABLE BOWEL SYNDROME
and
BLOATED STOMACH

These are probably the two conditions that I treat more than any other. I would estimate that more than half the patients I've treated over the years will have had one or both of these problems. In every case they will have made numerous trips to their GP and probably to the hospital for tests, and in most cases they will have been put on medication. As with all the people I see neither their doctors nor their medication has been of much use, otherwise they would not have turned up at my clinic looking for the answer. Having treated and cured many thousands of patients over the years I have proven that these two conditions are simply caused by active yeast fermenting when it is fed on sugar. You will find all the help you need to make a full recovery on pages 66 - 73. Let us now look at some letters from patients that suffered with these problems before coming to Health Scan.

The first letter is from a lady in Guernsey. Note that her hospital specialist said food had **nothing** to do with her condition.
Can you imagine what this poor lady had to go through for years before she found the answer at Health Scan?

Mrs B from Guernsey
"When I came to see you 3 months ago I was completely at the end of my tether. I was diagnosed with Colitis two years ago and from that moment on my life went downhill. My hospital specialist said food had nothing to do with my condition and I

131

underwent test after test without an answer. I had terrible stomach pains and some days I was on the toilet every half-hour missing quite a few days and weeks off work. I felt myself getting more and more depressed as it seemed everything I tried made no difference. You were my last hope and I can't thank you enough. Since my test with you I feel great, my life has changed around and I can now look forward to a brighter future."

The next letter is from a guy in his early twenties. These are the most precious years of all and a time when he should be out enjoying himself. A single food intolerance test has now allowed him to do that.

Mr W from Leeds

"I came to see you in July and you diagnosed certain foods that were making me feel unwell and ruining my life. Since my scan I have stopped getting the bloated stomach and I can honestly say that I feel like a new person. I am performing better at work and I am so much more interested in getting out and socialising. I really can't thank you enough for your help."

Our next letter is another Daily Express case.
It's been seven years since they and I got a copy of this letter, it's not too late you can still reach me at: **intolerance@healthscan.co.uk**

Oh!...and notice the increase in libido this guy enjoyed, this happens all the time.

Mr C from Essex

"As promised I have also sent a copy of this letter to The Daily Express. I am 29 years old and until recently a serving member of the Royal Air Force. In recent years I started to suffer with severe Irritable Bowel Syndrome and seeing an article in the Express about your work I came to see you. The test was quite

straightforward, painless and very interesting indeed. On my train journey home I studied the results and it became simple to understand just why I was suffering. It is now some two months after my scan and I feel fantastic (not so good for my wife). As the results proved so successful in every way my wife (hoping to withstand me) has just been for a test also. Many of my family have taken a keen interest in your work and will be coming to see you shortly. Many thanks to you and The Daily Express for my happier and healthier life."

Our next letter shows very clearly just how little GP's in general know about I.B.S.

This patient was told that his condition was **incurable** and that the best he could hope for was to take pills for the rest of his life.
Ten weeks after his scan he wrote this letter to say he was cured.

Mr P from Surrey
"I had suffered with I.B.S. for about two years and on my last visit to my GP the advice I was given was that it was incurable and that I would have to be prepared to live with it. Having been prescribed endless tablets and now with a GP that had given up on me I decided to try and find an alternative solution. Since my scan 10 weeks ago I have been totally cured, it's just incredible. This has given me an improved quality of life enabling me to fully enjoy my social life and to start a new and very demanding job.
I am extremely grateful to you and have no hesitation in fully recommending your scan to anyone."

The next letter is from the mum of a little girl called Chelsea.
She had been undergoing treatment at Eastbourne District General Hospital for some two years before being cured with a **single** food intolerance test at Health Scan. *Note:* She was also discharged from hospital following her scan. I wonder how much taxpayer's

money went into **unsuccessfully** treating Chelsea over those two years. Surely the doctors and their management should be made to account for such wasteful expenditure of public funds. As I've said before it's impossible to calculate the vast amount of taxpayer's money that's **wasted** every year by the NHS in its feeble attempt to treat the 53 or more health problems that I easily cure with a **single** food intolerance test. Technology as used at Health Scan would free up billions of pounds each and every year. This money could be put to better use within the medical system and/or used elsewhere such as in education or in law & order. Not only would there be a vast saving of public money but even more importantly patients could get on with living healthy lives instead of sitting for wasteful and countless hours in draughty hospital corridors.

Mrs S from Sussex

"I'm writing to you regarding our daughter Chelsea, since having the Health Scan she has changed the way she eats and has made a full recovery. She has now been discharged from the hospital after having two years of tests without success. This health scan is something that we would recommend to anyone, we are so grateful for the help we have received and wish to thank you."

Our next letter about David and Epsom Hospital will highlight yet again just how bigoted **most** doctors are when they come up against Alternative Medicine. Even when I was proved to be right this particular consultant refused to accept it. The worst thing of all is that if David's parents had not brought him to Health Scan then David would probably have spent the rest of his life with this condition.

WHY DOCTORS DON'T MAKE YOU HEALTHY.

Mrs A of Surrey
"Earlier this year we brought our five year old son David to see you and you identified 17 foods that he should avoid. For the last year he'd suffered with very bad stomach cramps which began at around 2pm and 7pm each day, this made his and our lives unbearable as he was going to the toilet almost hourly. Within about 5 days of our visit to your clinic we noticed a dramatic improvement and within two weeks his symptoms had almost disappeared completely. It is now some five months since his scan and he appears to be totally 'CURED'. Two weeks ago we took David back to see his consultant at Epsom Hospital. We told the consultant of David's recovery and she said that she could see no scientific explanation for the sudden change in his health. She suggested that we put David back onto the foods which we had taken him off as this should make no difference. Within hours of eating the banned foods he was again curled up on the settee with the same old stomach cramps and diarrhoea. We have since returned to the items you said to avoid and he has returned to good health yet again. Thank you very much for your help, the difference it has made to David and to the rest of the family is immeasurable."

You will notice how David's doctor came up with that regular old favourite of medical objections when she said that she could find no **scientific** reason why foods should be the cause or answer to his problem. Since medicine began doctors have been hiding behind this particular quote when faced with something they do not understand or results that embarrass them.

There is after all an old saying that doctors bury their mistakes. First of all I doubt that this particular doctor has ever read up on food intolerance so how could she know how effective it is. When faced with one of her patients having been cured by such testing she then takes a negative attitude and by so doing advises incorrectly yet again. There is plenty of scientific material available to support food intolerance testing and if she had shown the slightest interest in her other patients future welfare then the least she could have done was to have picked up the phone and talked to me. The technology used at Health Scan has been licensed by the American Food & Drugs Administration who are the toughest licensing body in the world and I can assure David's doctor that such a licence would not have been granted had there not been ample **scientific** evidence produced.

Read the following letter from Alexander's mum and call me soft if you will but when I can stop a five year old's tummy from **"stinging"** it almost brings tears of joy to my eyes.

Mrs M from Surrey

"I brought my five year old son to see you at the beginning of February to be tested for food intolerance. For about 18 months previous to our visit Alexander had been suffering from tummy aches and other digestive complaints, which understandably made him miserable most of the time. On top of this he was prone to very silly and noisy behaviour with poor concentration and he could whinge for Britain. As some days were worse than others I felt sure that his problems must be food related. Within two or three days of his scan we noticed vast improvements in David's behaviour and his tummy pains and bloated stomach disappeared. Now three months down the line whinging is a thing of the past, he has much more stamina and I feel that my happy sunny child has been returned to me. David has had to do without some of his favourites like chips and chocolate but he readily accepts it as he doesn't want his 'tummy to sting again' Thank you very much for providing the answer to a problem that had us at our wit's end."

Our next letter shows how this scan helps in other ways also as this girl was able to concentrate much better on her schoolwork once her I.B.S. was cured. What chance do children or adults have of concentrating on their studies if they are unhealthy?

Mrs R from Surrey

"I am writing to inform you of my daughter's **GOOD NEWS** *since her scan on October 16th. Having cut out all the bad foods her I.B.S. has cleared and she has not had a single problem with it since, we are absolutely delighted with the results. Fortunately she has now been able to catch up with most of her schoolwork and has had a fair attempt at her mock GCSE's. Thank you for all your help and guidance."*

Again I say it, if these doctors whose patients I am curing really had the best interests of their **other** patients at heart instead of their own pathetic sense of self-importance then the least they should have done was to pick up the phone for a chat. Or is it me just being silly here…Am I expecting too much?

Our next letter highlights yet again the nonsense that is the NHS. This patient was cured within a week of a scan after **15 years** of unsuccessful treatment under god knows how many consultants and other so called *(and costly)* specialists.

Mr K from Hertfordshire

"It is now 6 weeks since I had my Health Scan, within the first week my I.B.S. disappeared and this is after 15 years of useless NHS consultations and treatment. My symptoms return if I try and eat the forbidden foods. I can now say without reservation that by following the diet I have become incredibly healthy and far more energetic. Thank you for all your help, I shall of course give you all the publicity I can."

Mr K above had suffered with I.B.S. for 15 years but our next patient suffered with it for more than **30 years**. Can you imagine that? He went through thirty years of unnecessary pain whilst paying money to drug companies for useless and possibly harmful drugs.

"Thank you so much for curing me of I.B.S. as I had suffered with it for over 30 years and had tried every medicine available but nothing worked. Your work is truly miraculous."

I also have a letter from ***Mrs S of Surrey***. I cured her stomach pain and bloating with a single scan after she'd suffered with them **all her life!** You would logically think that under the circumstances she could now bring **and win** a claim for damages against the NHS for the **unnecessary** suffering she endured throughout those years. She says her bowel consultant was very interested in my work.

It's been 7 years now, maybe he'll ring tomorrow!

Chapter **27**

LETHARGY & DEPRESSION

SEROXAT is an anti-depressive drug widely prescribed by the medical profession. I.T.V. News stated on 10th June 2003 that Seroxat was **'unlicensed'** and that it reportedly caused suicidal tendencies in teenagers. Having watched a TV documentary about Seroxat on BBC's Panorama programme on the 12th May 2003 I will now list the side effects that were reported by the patient's unfortunate enough to be taking it. You can draw your own conclusions:

Anxiety.
Confusion.
Dilated pupils.
Electric shock sensations in the brain.
Hot flushes.
Lack of concentration.
Lethargy.
Loss of balance.
Loss of feeling and emotions.
Major weight gain.
Nausea.
Panic attacks.
Restlessness.
Shivering.
Sleeplessness.
Suicidal tendencies.
Sweating.
Violent aggression.
Violent nightmares.

WHY DOCTORS DON'T MAKE YOU HEALTHY.

So a patient with depression visits their doctor and is put on this stuff, sorry am I missing something here? I thought medication was **supposed** to make you better, not worse! *(All the above information was taken from the BBC website immediately after the programme)* On Tuesday 30th March 2004 G.M.T.V. News reported that one in every three patients seen by a G.P. are prescribed anti-depressants. G.Ps say that they have no other choice. If you think **SEROXAT** is bad then take a look at the side effects of another commonly used anti-depressant called **PROZAC**:

(Source/Internet)

Aggressive or violent behaviour.
Blank staring.
Blurred vision or pressure behind the eyes.
Breathing or lung problems.
Burning or tingling in extremities.
Chills or cold sweats.
Confusion.
Cravings for alcohol sweets and other substances, or drinking large amounts of alcohol coffee or other caffeinated drinks.
Deceitfulness.
Diabetes or hypoglycaemia.
Dizziness.
Extreme fatigue.
Falsely accusing others of abuse, family members or acquaintances.
Hair loss.
Headaches.
Heart fluttering.
Hyperactivity.
Impulsive behaviour with no concern about consequences.
Inability to detect dreams from reality.

Inability to discontinue use of drug and increasing own dose.
Inability to feel guilt or cry.
Inability to see any alternatives in situations.
Insomnia.
Loss of appetite.
Loss of spirituality...feeling 'possessed' or that something evil is inside.
Lowered immune system.
Mania.
Memory impairment.
Mood swings...altered personality.
Muscle tremors...loss of co-ordination.
Muscle twitching or contractions.
Muscle weakness.
Nausea.
No desire to be touched.
No emotions.
Numbness in various body parts. Legs go numb and right out from under patient; or sexual organs go numb making orgasm impossible.
Paranoia.
Psychosis.
Pulling away from loved ones and others.
Rash.
Seizures or convulsions.
Self-destructive behaviour and suicidal ideation.
Shaking, jitteriness.
Sweating.
Swelling and/or pain in joints.
Symptoms of mania, i.e.: inability to sit still or restlessness racing thoughts, acting silly or giddy (like a teenager again) sexual promiscuity leading to unwanted pregnancy or divorce irresponsibility, wild spending sprees, gambling, criminal behaviour, shoplifting, embezzling, stealing, hostility etc.

Tongue numbness and slurred speech.
Unusual energy surges at times producing super human strength.
Vivid and violent dreams.
Wanting to ram other cars or driving irrationally.
Weight gain or weight loss.

Ah!...Personally I think the patient might be better off sticking with depression than risking the side effects of this wonderful medication. In severe cases of depression Electro-Convulsive therapy is used and if that fails then it's almost certainly a one way ticket to the mental hospital. When a patient reports symptoms of lethargy many doctors will test the Thyroid Gland to see if it's under active. If this is found to be the case then the patient is put on a lifetime course of Thyroxine. Great for the drug companies but not so good for the patient and/or the NHS *(taxpayer)* that has to pay for it.

But stop for a moment doc!

Q.   What runs your Thyroid Gland?

A.   Your brain!

Yes!...That's right doc!...Well done!

So why not get the brain working properly and maybe then it will run the Thyroid Gland properly! It might seem a strange thing to say doc but I hope it's not too hard to get your head around the fact that if you **DON'T** poison your brain then it will work properly. Not only will it run your body properly for the **FIRST** time in your life but your energy and concentration levels also increase dramatically.

WHY DOCTORS DON'T MAKE YOU HEALTHY.

Ah!…um!…quick….lets change the subject!

Let's look at some letters while the doc is thinking about that.

Our first letter is from a Mum whose 9-year-old daughter had suffered with severe lack of energy the whole of her short life. The medical profession could not help but I cured her in a few months. Note once again how the child's GP was not interested or supportive with regard to her condition or her food.

Mrs T from Hertfordshire
*"My daughter's main problems were Wheat and Lactose and we gradually took them away from her. I went to my GP to ask for assistance with this diet but unfortunately he was not very supportive. This made me feel quite angry as he had not been able to solve her tiredness **in nine years**. His attitude made me even more determined to try the new diet. We started seeing results within weeks, she started looking brighter and the dark lines under her eyes were going. Now she has lots more energy and is a happy normal child, thank you so much for your help."*

Again our next letter highlights the problems that mint in toothpaste often causes. Although this wasn't the only problem that this patient had, it was by far the biggest.

Miss C from Surrey
*"I have always felt lethargic, forgetful, dizzy and nauseous. Although I have been tested many times for many things the tests always came back clear. I had just about given up when I came to Health Scan. Within days of cutting everything out I noticed improvements, **it's so wonderful that I don't have to take pills anymore** or do any more tests. A simple thing like changing my toothpaste has made such a massive difference to my health.*

I can't believe that all those foods I ate over the years were just making the situation worse. I am more positive and productive at work now and my home life is much happier too. I find it amazing that after all these years of suffering that there is absolutely nothing wrong with me anymore and it was so simple. I don't think I ever felt so healthy I just wish I'd had a food intolerance test years ago."

The young lady in our next letter made numerous expensive visits to her private doctor. (*She had obviously lost faith in the NHS*) Wow!...What a specialist!...The best he could do was to take her money and advise her to take up Yoga.

If this weren't so serious it could be a joke!

Mrs W from Middx
"I had been suffering from increasing bouts of fatigue and a debilitating lack of energy since the birth of my son 10 years ago. Having visited my private doctor numerous times over the 10 years he could only advise me to take up Yoga. Since having my Health Scan I no longer suffer the overwhelming feeling of exhaustion and I have an increased level of energy that I thought I would never experience again."

The lady in our next letter feels that this testing should be free for all on the NHS, now that would be good but while the drug companies are so powerful I can't really see it happening.

Although you never know I might get a call from Mr Blair or Mr Bush one of these days...Yeh!...Yeh!

I've probably got more chance of being struck by lightening.

Mrs C from Kent

"It's been 4 weeks since I came to see you and the benefits are many and marvellous. I now feel a vitality I thought I'd lost forever years ago. It's like waking up and coming out of a fog.
I used to feel so lethargic and that frustrated me because I desperately wanted to have more energy. I used to think I must be suffering from S.A.D. (Seasonal Affective Disorder – It's a type of winter Depression) or M.E. (Myalgic Encephalomyelitis). Now I no longer sleep in the afternoons as I have so much energy to do things instead of slumping in the chair and feeling sorry for myself. I am so glad I had the test done and very grateful to you for showing me the way to a happier healthier life. I think this testing should be free on the NHS so that everyone can have a chance to become healthy."

Here! Here!

Our last quote is from *Mrs E from Norfolk.*
She suffered most of her life from panic attacks and severe depression and all she could look forward to was many more years of useless medication.

If this lady had been born 50 years earlier she would most certainly have been considered a prime candidate for incarceration into a mental hospital. She is now **drug free** and living a happy healthy life. *"Thank you for giving me my life back, your work is incredible."*

(Source: BBC News Friday 20th June 2003)
The Committee on Safety of Medicines has ruled that the anti-depressant drug SEROXAT should not now be prescribed to under 18's as it was not licensed to be used in such cases.
(Maybe it was only licensed to be used to poison patients that were over 18?)

The report says that an estimated 8,000 under 18-year olds were on this drug. Approximately four million prescriptions *(now there's a nice little earner)* had been written over the previous twelve months.

***

Anti-depressants are taken by 3.5 million people every day in the UK.   (Source: Sunday Express 12th December 2004)

The number of prescriptions issued has risen from 1 million in 1993 to 13 million in 2004.
(Source: GMTV News 30th March 2004)

The government agency responsible for regulating drugs admitted that they do **NOT** look at all data on anti-depressants i.e. Prozac but rely heavily on **summaries** from clinical trials.
(Source: Sunday Express 12th December 2004)

To the best of my knowledge drug companies either carryout their own trials on drugs that they produce or they pay others to do them. So any summary of the results can be as brief and **non-informative** as they wish because drug companies have no legal obligation to reveal the results of such trials. Surely the time must come when a completely independent body *(if that's possible)* will be given the task of monitoring such dangerous products.

Chapter **28**

MIGRAINE / HEADACHES

There are some 23 million sufferers of migraine/headaches in the U.S. and 92% are women (Source: Internet). I've treated vast numbers of migraine/headache sufferers and have yet to find one that I have not cured with a **single** food intolerance test. As I mentioned before if you give your brain a problem then it gives you one!...That sounds fair to me. You could poison your brain with alcohol and be **sure** of a headache or you could do it with food and get one also. If your brain **does not want** a drug be it alcohol or chicken it will tell you in so many different ways, pain is just one of those ways.

Remember: It's your **brain** that runs your body!...Not your taste buds or stomach.

If you deliberately poisoned your brain with drugs it didn't want then you would expect problems. Well you're doing that (but not deliberately) with food every day so don't be surprised when your brain gives you **pain** in return.

Our first two migraine letters are from patients that suffered for many years with **Cluster Headaches / Migraines**. The first letter was written only four months after her scan. A reporter at The Daily Express got a copy yet again...But hey!...It's only been 7 years...I'm sure they'll call soon.

Mrs A from Sussex

"It is with much pleasure that I'm writing to you to say that after my visit to your clinic and following your instructions I can now say that my 'CLUSTER HEADACHES' and regular 'MIGRAINE' are things of the past. I really appreciate waking in the morning with a clear head. Without your system I am sure I would never have found the cause of my problem. Thank you for all the help you have given me."

Our next letter shows yet again what a total nonsense our so-called health system is. The best this lady could hope for from her **HIGHLY PAID AND EXPENSIVELY TRAINED** Neurologist after 20 years of suffering with migraine was to spend the rest of her life financing drug companies with pill popping of **Imigran** and other expensive and pointless drugs.

Mrs T of Nottingham

"Since my Health Scan 3 months ago I felt I must write and let you know how much better I am feeling. I have suffered with migraine for over 20 years and recently on a daily basis (cluster migraines). I have tried Acupuncture, Reflexology, Iridology, Chinese herbs and a host of other natural remedies to no avail. Recently I consulted a Neurologist and was prescribed tablets to relax me and Imigran to take when needed. A friend told me about Health Scan so I thought what have I got to lose. It revealed a major intolerance to Wheat, Yeast and some dairy products and amazingly within a week of cutting them out my migraine had gone. I only wish that I had known about Health Scan years ago, I would certainly recommend it to everyone. If only the National Health Service would look at alternative treatment and save themselves billions of pounds on the pills they prescribe."

WHY DOCTORS DON'T MAKE YOU HEALTHY.

Nice letter Mrs T. Someone somewhere should be answerable for ruining 20 years of her life with inadequate treatment when all along the answer was so simple. Surely Mrs T and all the other millions of patients that suffer unnecessarily should have a right to claim for damages against the NHS or the so-called *'private specialists'* that continue to rake in vast sums of money for little or no results. Just how do you put a price on ruining twenty years of a person's life?

The man in our next letter didn't feel that he needed testing as he considered himself reasonably healthy, he only came to the clinic to accompany his wife who was having hers. Brian decided to have a scan on the spur of the moment after reading my testimonial letters and after listening to me explaining my work. As he watched me scanning his wife he realised at long last that he had found someone who could really help him as he had been suffering with headaches for many years. Isn't it strange how people can live with such things as headaches and yet consider themselves healthy. Brian had been through the slog of conventional medicine and had long given up hope of finding a cure. As with our previous letter Brian had also tried numerous other therapies without success: Aromatherapy, Homeopathy and Herbal remedies etc. All the patients I've treated over the years had at least been through conventional medicine and a high proportion of them will also have been to numerous alternative health specialists as Brian did. The reason that none of these other treatments worked was that in **all** cases the specialist was trying to treat the symptoms, whereas I find the cause.

Remember doc: When you find the **cause** of a problem and you remove it, guess what!...**The problem disappears!**...Simple eh!

So if you haven't got a **problem** you don't need **medication**.
(Not that it works anyway!)

Brian from Cornwall

"It is now 4 months since I had my scan with you and the results are amazing. After many years of living with headaches it was like a miracle to find such a simple cure. I had been to loads of doctors and rather than live on pills I just put up with the headaches. I also tried most other forms of alternative treatment and they didn't work either. It's hard to believe that something as simple as basic everyday food was causing my problem all along. Thank you very much for your help, I have of course recommended you to my family and friends some of whom have been to you already."

Our next letter shows a **cure** for **severe headaches and migraine** in just 3 months. Quite a list of other health problems cleared up also.

Mrs T from Birmingham

"It is now 3 months since I was tested and I am delighted to tell you how well the scan has worked for me. I came to you with a history of severe headaches and migraine, high blood pressure weight problems, acidity and back spasms. I am pleased to let you know that these have all now cleared up and my blood pressure is normal once again. I thank you for everything and wish you all the success you deserve."

The next letter shows a **very** happy 61-year old lady that has not only got rid of her headaches but has also found a **major increase** in her libido.

Miss A from Surrey

"Having removed all the bad foods my constant headaches have gone completely but there is an added 'unexpected' bonus as my libido has increased dramatically and wow!...What a difference

that has made to my social life, I feel and act like a 20 year old again, thank you so much your scanning is fantastic."

The following extracts from three letters highlight once again just how easy it is to become healthy. You will see how one of the patients was quite sceptical before coming to Health Scan. This is of course only to be expected especially if a person has not come via a recommendation. I know it is hard to believe that such suffering is so simple to cure especially if you've had a lifetime of tramping around dark and dingy hospital corridors looking for an answer, especially if you've seen numerous so-called **'top'** migraine specialists. How then one might ask can a person who's not a doctor actually help? Remember that **every single one** of the many thousands of patients I've cured had already **been** to see doctors. People are just brain washed by a lifetime of being told that doctors cure people; most adults **and doctors** know that is not true.

Mrs W from Wales

"It has been just over a month since I saw you and what a difference this month has made. As you know I had been suffering from migraine for many years but now there gone. Overall I feel my body is in great shape and I feel super healthy, I don't know how to thank you enough for your help and kindness. I only wish I had come to see you 8 years ago when my migraine first started."

Mrs S from Norfolk

"May I say how delighted I am with the improvements to my condition since having a Health Scan, not only have my severe headaches disappeared but I have also regained control of my stomach and waistline. I have been recommending Health Scan to friends and relatives on the grounds of its efficiency speed and non-invasive nature which in my opinion makes it a treatment far

preferable to any other methods available either privately or on the NHS."

Miss R from Newcastle
"I visited you on the 25th November 1998 as I was suffering from very bad migraine and had been for many years. I have to admit that I was quite sceptical as to whether my headaches were due to my diet but I can now honestly say that since visiting you I have been 100% migraine free. Thank you very much for helping me with this problem, I also feel much better in myself and have a great deal more energy."

The first of our final two letters is from a lady that suffered with migraine for the whole of her life until she came to Health Scan. Note how her symptoms came back again when she cheated and ate the forbidden foods at Xmas, if this isn't **proof** of food being the **cause** and **solution** then what is?

As you will see the lady in our second letter made an incredible recovery after being treated **without success** for some 3 years by her hospital and GP. She also sent her G.P. Dr Steer a copy of this letter.

It's only been 7 years...maybe Dr Steer will ring tomorrow!

Mrs W from Surrey
"I have suffered migraine and digestive problems all my life. Amazingly within a month or so of coming off the poisonous foods my headaches, digestive problem and mood swings had gone. Unfortunately I relapsed over Xmas and my symptoms came back so that made me even more determined to stick to my diet."

Mrs A from Hants

"During the last three years I have suffered from a lot of headaches and a number of unexplained vomiting attacks. I had several investigations for these but no cause was found, my doctor diagnosed migraine and suggested that I experiment with diet. At this point luckily I came to you and found the answer in a simple one-hour test, incredible but true. My blood pressure has also returned to normal and I now sleep much better."

In the early months of the year 2000 I carried out free clinical trials on nine migraine sufferers who were members of a charity run national migraine organisation. The results were incredibly successful but that was as far as it went. What I would like to bring to your attention is the fact that there were 35 other **so called** specialist clinics listed on the back of their brochure.

I wonder how many hopefuls have sat in **their** corridors over the years, I wonder to how many of them were cured. To the best of my knowledge not one of these other clinics will be carrying out food intolerance testing. I don't suppose many of them will even be discussing food with their patients much less testing it. God knows how much these places cost to run each year probably millions of pounds of taxpayer's money that could well be put to better use. It's the same old argument lets face it. These organisations only make money from people that are unhealthy just as doctors and drug companies do, so from a business point of view why would they want to cure them? If they were to acknowledge that food intolerance was the solution to migraine and cure their members in this way then they would not only lose them but in time they would also lose their jobs.

Chapter **29**

MULTIPLE SCLEROSIS (M.S.)

I get very few requests for help with M.S. but when these patients phone my clinic for advice I always tell them that I cannot cure their condition.

But I can help them to feel better. Following a scan their brain will not be poisoned with harmful drugs called food. As a result it will then be able to run their body far better and to cope more efficiently with their M.S. condition.

The following letter is an example of such a case.

Miss L from Hampshire.
"I thought I would write and let you know how delighted I am with the effect that eliminating my problem foods has had on my health. Since visiting you six months ago and sticking to the diet my M.S. symptoms have been kept at bay and I feel much brighter. I am already recommending you to my friends for other ailments and I would not hesitate to recommend you to others."

Chapter **30**

WEIGHT

I get a great deal of success with weight loss and in my experience it's the **water** in our body that causes our weight to increase. Yes I know all the doctors and books tell us to drink lots of water if we want to lose weight; well if that advice was correct all you ladies and gents out there would be super slim. Okay!...Let me explain: If we took the water out of our body we'd be a pile of dust, you could hold it in your hand. Water makes up about 90% of our body weight and water is the **only** substance that absorbs into the cells/wall of the stomach. All other items are broken down **in** the stomach and pass into the intestines before being absorbed into the body. That's why so many people put weight on around the stomach, its just water being absorbed as it would into a sponge. What actually happens is that we fill up these stomach cells and the water then passes into other cells through osmosis and on into other parts of the body. When you drink a glass of water it doesn't all come out the other end, try measuring it sometime. So, if **some** of the water doesn't come out then it **must** still be in our body, and it is, and you know how heavy water is. I know we are told to drink two or three litres of water a day to flush out our toxins and to cleanse our Liver and Kidneys. That's fine if you have a medical condition that warrants all that water otherwise keep your liquid intake low and watch your weight reduce in the coming months. More weight will be lost if you follow my advice *(in this book)* properly and/or have a food intolerance test as your brain will work better. It can then run your metabolism better and deal more effectively with your future intake of water as well as the water that has already built up in your body.

Q. How much water should we drink a day?

WHY DOCTORS DON'T MAKE YOU HEALTHY.

A. The simple rule is to drink **small** amounts of water or fluids of any kind as the less you put in the less you will absorb and therefore the less you will have to lose.

But don't be silly and dehydrate yourself as that will only cause further problems. Sip a glass of water instead of drinking the whole thing in one go, make it last half a day, a mouthful of water will quench your thirst just the same as a glass full.

Think about it this way. If I were a farmer and I wanted to make a lot of money when I sold my cow at market I'd try to make her as heavy as possible because I get paid by **weight**. So I'd put lots of salt into her food and I'd give her a **salt-lick** to suck on, the salt would make her thirsty and she'd drink lots of water. Then on would go the weight and my bank manager would be very happy. You only have to think how small a piece of meat shrinks to when cooked to know that it's full of water, well that's all we are just a piece of meat. I've actually heard of farmers who put a hosepipe down the cow's throat and fill its stomach full of water before it goes in to be weighed for selling.

Sweat is nature's way of losing excess water and salt from the body so if you sweat then this is good news if you want to lose weight. Don't drink 2 litres of water a day and put it all back in. If you sweat a lot when playing sport then pour water onto your head and back to cool down rather than drinking vast amounts of it.

Remember to keep your salt intake to a minimum as salt will just make you thirsty.

Note:

Doctor Robert Atkins the world famous author of weight loss books made millions of pounds advising others on how to stay slim. At his death in April 2003 he was clinically obese weighing some 258lbs. That's 18.5 stone or 111kgs and his books are still selling in great numbers today. **Funny old world!**

Probably 75% of our testimonial letters mention weight loss to some degree or other. Even if patients don't actually come in with a weight problem weight will still fall off if they've got it to lose. I could fill this book with patient's comments on weight loss but I will only show extracts from a few letters where people have lost considerable weight.

Mr A & Mr T from Malaga

"It is with great joy that we write to tell you how wonderful we feel since we had our computerised food intolerance tests. Since the test I have lost a stone and a half and my headaches have gone completely. Bill has lost over 2 stone and he doesn't get out of breath like he used to. We are really enjoying life to the full and we thank you sincerely for all your help."

Mrs H from Birmingham

"Just to let you know that I am 6 weeks down the road from testing and feel wonderful. I am 1 stone lighter and look great."

Mrs S from Norfolk

"I visited you for a Health Scan some 4 months ago and I can truthfully say it is best money I have ever spent. I cut out all the troublesome foods and have lost just over one stone in weight, my weight has now levelled off to what it should be and I feel like a new woman."

Mr K from Bradford

"Since my visit to you I have lost 1 stone in weight without feeling hungry. I feel and look good now for the first time in many years, thank you so much."

Miss P from Hull

"In February I attended your clinic for a food intolerance test considerably overweight and hoping for some magical cure. Well I can honestly say I have found it as I have now lost 2 stone without really doing much except eating the right foods. I am feeling very well now and wish to thank you sincerely for all your help."

Chapter 31

TOURETTE SYNDROME

To give this condition its full name it's Gilles de la Tourette's Syndrome.

I have only ever treated two children suffering with this rare condition.

Case 1: A 10-year-old boy was flown from Stockholm to see if I could help with his Tourette's. This condition is very rare indeed, the patient will make sudden involuntary movements and often shout obscenities. (Peter Sellers once played the role of Doctor Strangelove, a man with this condition in the film of the same name). This lad's condition developed when he was about 4 years old, he was brought to see me by his mum and grandparents. I had cured his grandparents some months earlier of migraine etc.

When they first asked if I could help with their grandson's condition I said that I did not know as I had never been asked to treat Tourette's before so I could not say if food intolerance was the answer. This is what Mosby's Medical dictionary tells us about Tourette Syndrome. Mosby's is the bible of the medical world. Doctors refer to it all the time to read up on details of various health problems and possible treatments.

(Gilles de la Tourette, French neurologist born 1857)
An abnormal condition characterised by facial grimaces, tics and involuntary arm and shoulder movements. In adolescence the condition worsens; the child may grunt, snort, and shout involuntarily.

Coprolalia (The excessive use of obscene language) *often develops, affecting judgement of the condition by the family and society. In adulthood the condition usually does not worsen; it comes and goes. Recently, treatment with dopamine antagonists has been found to be very effective, demonstrating an organic cause for this syndrome.*

Yes!... And that **organic** cause looks very much like food intolerance!

After 150 years I may just have found the answer!

The lad had been treated at several so-called specialist hospitals since the onset of his condition. Now at the age of ten the best they could offer was to put him on a **lifelong** course of drugs for treatment of schizophrenia, his parents adamantly refused to allow this. Having scanned the lad I am now 99.9% certain that I have found the cause of his condition as he had the biggest intolerance to **Wheat and Cheese** that I have seen for many years. And what did he eat for breakfast, dinner and tea? **Bread/Cheese/Pasta and Pizzas!** He ate no (*so-called*) proper meals he just filled himself up with these items every single day. Obviously mum and dad never thought that bread cheese and pasta could be harmful so they were happy for him to eat them whenever and wherever he wished. If any of you reading this are suffering with Tourette's or know of someone that does then do please email me for an update on the outcome of this case as the lad's parents have agreed to keep me up-dated via email.

Case 2: Coincidentally shortly after I had scanned the lad in case 1 above I flew out to Abu Dhabi in the UAE to scan this next lad. This boy was 12 years old and had suffered from the condition most of his life. The world's finest doctors (*or should I say the worlds most expensive doctors*) had written him off as incurable they said that he would have to live with his condition. Within a few months of his scan he had virtually made a full recovery.

The lad showed a very high intolerance to most of the vegetables he was eating and to very little else except mint. He and his whole family were vegetarian and even when his parents saw their son's dramatic improvement with their own eyes they still couldn't accept the fact that these **healthy** foods had been the cause of such a problem all these years. Mum is a totally obsessed vegetarian and to this day she has insisted on keeping her son on a few of the **healthy** vegetables to which he was intolerant, otherwise he would, I'm sure, have made a full recovery.

Chapter **32**

UNUSUAL CASES

Talk about coals to Newcastle! One of Europe's biggest drug companies with their head office in West London sent me patients from their own medical department on a regular basis for many years.

Two sister's came in for a scan they both suffered with severe migraine, one also had IBS. They both showed a major intolerance to yeast and mint. One of the sisters was employed by the pharmaceutical company mentioned above to research a cure for IBS. In both cases their migraine was caused by mint toothpaste which was made by this same drug company that employed one of them!

A first year **medical student** came to me with severe arthritis. It's no wonder she had such pain in her body she had a massive intolerance to wheat, yeast and mint.

A *(lady)* director of an international weight loss company came to see me in Harley Street to lose weight.

A lady came in with **severe** skin problems on her hands; her biggest intolerance was to **cod** fish. She worked in a fish and chip shop.

A professional golfer came for a scan to try and identify why his back 9 holes were **always** worse than his front 9. The two bananas he religiously ate half way through his game were the cause.

A lady that worked in a launderette: She always suffered with inflamed and itchy hands after her day at work. When she didn't work she was fine. Obviously she had been for numerous allergy tests that included testing for washing powder etc. It turned out to be the newspaper she read in her break as she had a massive intolerance to newsprint. She only read newspapers at work, she didn't bother with them on her days off.

A lady golfer that suffered with a skin rash on her neck. It **only** happened when she played golf. She was intolerant to the leather handle on her golf club.

An elderly lady that had severe migraine for a great many years. It **always** started late on a Friday night and cleared by Monday or Tuesday. For as long as she could remember she and her husband visited a local restaurant and ate fish and chips on a Friday night. She had a **major** intolerance to Haddock…her favourite fish.

All of the above had intolerance to other foods etc …but it's interesting how sometimes the **major** cause of a problem is not so obvious.

Often when I'm scanning a patient if their partner is present I would say how this test will make her/him 20 years younger.
One day I was scanning a lady and I said this to her husband.
His wife was 60 years old and I said how I would make her 40 again. He quickly replied:

"Could I have two 20 year olds instead?"

Chapter **33**

ROYALTY and HEALTH SCAN

Yes!…They're human too you know!
Can't go into any detail, sorry!
I'd very much like to but I'd better not as I won't get my Knighthood!

Here's an envelope though. Note the postmark:

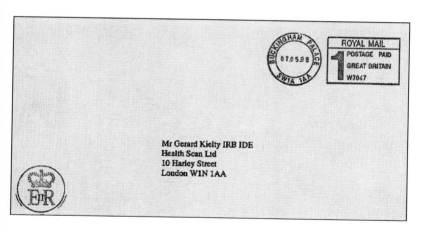

Each year I travel several times to Abu Dhabi in The Middle East where I scan Sheikhs and their families, to date I have scanned about 200 of them. I have also scanned about 60 of the Saudi Royal family. It all started when a few of them came to see me in Harley Street and as they recovered from their health problems it just snowballed. The reason I mention this is that if my work was not successful do you think that the richest people in the world would want me to treat them. Their doctors have been getting very rich on these families for the last 50 years or so since the oil started flowing but they have failed in so many ways to cure them. These Royal and Ruling families are so happy that they have found Health Scan and that they have found a way to become healthy at long last without doctors or drugs.

PART 4

WHY DOCTORS DON'T MAKE YOU HEALTHY

34

MERCURY IN AMALGAM

Now, what about **Mercury in Amalgam** that dentists have been filling our teeth with for the past 50 years or more?

Mercury is the most **toxic** metal known to man, it's even more toxic than arsenic and they put it four inches from our brain.

There's masses of clinical trials been done over the years that **prove** beyond doubt that mercury leaks from our teeth and passes through our gums and into our bloodstream and nervous system. But nothing ever gets done about it. The powers that be refuse to accept results of any kind which show that mercury actually leaks from our teeth. There may also be a lot more healthy pensioners around if they hadn't gone through life with a mouthful of mercury. I sometimes wonder if that is why so many of our parents had false teeth all those years ago. Did dentists realise their mistake and try to reverse the process in those early days? You don't hear of many people having **all** their teeth out these days do you?

I'd also love to remove the fillings of a group of M.S. and Mental Patients to see to what extent they recovered over a given period of a year or so.

The following report *(which has been paraphrased here)* was written by a dentist.

WHY DOCTORS DON'T MAKE YOU HEALTHY.

Scientifically Proven Facts about Mercury and Amalgam

Teeth are a living tissue and are part of our body and they have a massive communication via the blood, lymph and nerves with the rest of the body.

Mercury from amalgam fillings is the single greatest source of dietary Mercury for the general population (W.H.O. criteria 118. 1991). Mercury from amalgam is absorbed and retained in the body at a rate of at least 1 microgram per surface of amalgam filling per day. Mercury from amalgam will migrate through the tooth. The rate that this occurs at is increased if a gold crown is placed over a tooth filled with amalgam.

Mercury vapour is the main way that mercury comes out of amalgam and Mercury vapour is absorbed at a rate of about 80% through the lungs into the arterial blood.

There is NO safe level of mercury vapour.

Mercury comes out of silver amalgam fillings at a rate of 10mcg/day. After chewing, the raised mercury vapour levels will remain raised for at least another 90 minutes.
New high copper amalgams release mercury 50 times faster than the old amalgams. Mercury from amalgam comes out at a rate that can easily cause toxic mercury poisoning.

Mercury release is increased by:

1. An increase in temperature
2. Friction
3. An increase in electrical currents

Mercury is cytotoxic. That is to say it kills cells.

Mercury from amalgam binds to – SH (sulphydryl) groups. These exist in almost every enzymatic process in the body. Mercury from amalgam will thus have the potential of disturbing all metabolic processes.

Mercury from amalgam will enter the body as;

- Elemental mercury
- Inorganic mercury
- Vapour
- Charged mercury ions

Mercury is the most toxic metal we know. However, Methyl Mercury is more toxic than Elemental Mercury and Mercury from amalgam is methylated in the mouth and many other areas of the body.

Mercury from amalgam is stored preferentially in the Pituitary Gland and Hypothalamus and causes long term low level mercury poisoning – Micro Mercurialism. Micro Mercurialism is principally characterised by neurological symptoms where Mercury from amalgam crosses and destroys the blood brain barrier. It is then transported along the axons of nerve fibres. Mercury from amalgams is implicated in the pathogenesis of Alzheimer's Disease. Generally brain levels of Mercury are in a direct linear proportion to the number of surfaces of amalgam fillings in the mouth. Mercury from amalgam is also absorbed by the kidneys the liver and the brain.

Mercury from amalgam causes kidney damage causing a 50% reduction in kidney filtration within 2 months of placement.

Mercury from amalgam may be stored in every cell in the body. Each area affected will produce its own set of symptoms.

For example, Mercury from amalgam binds to haemoglobin in the red blood cells thus reducing there oxygen carrying capacity.

Mercury from amalgam is stored preferentially in the foetus and infant before the mother. In fact Mercury from amalgam is stored in the breast milk and the foetus up to eight times more than the mother's tissue.

Mercury from amalgam will cause single strand breaks in DNA which severely reduces the reproductive function.

Mercury from amalgam rapidly depletes the immune system and can induce a number of Auto-Immune Diseases.

Mercury from amalgam will cause an increase in the number and severity of allergies.

Mercury from amalgam damages blood vessels and reduces blood supply to the tissues. (micro-angiopathies)

Amalgam fillings produce electrical currents that are themselves injurious to health. These currents are measurable in Micro Amps. The Central Nervous System (Brain) operates in the range of Nano Amps that are One Thousand times 'less' than a Micro Amp.

Mercury from amalgam will induce antibiotic resistance in bacteria in the mouth and gastrointestinal tract.

Mercury levels in the body cannot be assessed by either blood or urine levels.

It is a travesty of arrogance and ignorance that the dental associations continue to promote the use of this poison.

As dentists, the thing we do most often is fill teeth. Really what we are doing is placing inorganic material into living tissue.
As such we are in reality Implant Surgeons and each 'filling' is an implant. It is very rare that dentistry considers the systematic effects of such treatments and I would suggest that when amalgam is placed the systematic effects are **NEVER** considered. If they were then every implant of this material would constitute intentional criminal poisoning!

THERE IS 'NO' SAFE FORM OF MERCURY

...............(End of Dentist's Report)...............

Wow!...Now there's something to think about.

I remember watching a BBC documentary on this very subject several years ago. A great deal of such evidence and support data was delivered by hand to the headquarters of The British Dental Association. The whole thing was filmed as the files were handed over and a response was requested in due course. A month or two later the film crew and report specialists returned and were invited in. The camera showed three or four BDA directors sitting behind a huge desk. They were asked for their comments on the files that had been previously handed in.

"Which files?" They asked.

The files in front of you on your desk replied the interviewer.

"Oh!...We haven't had time to look at those." Was the sarcastic reply. They were told they would get a reply **when and if** their people had time to read the reports.

Guess what!...I never heard anymore!...I don't suppose anyone else did either.

If there is an element of truth in the dentist's report that you have just read *(and personally my money is on the dentist)* then why does no one in the BDA or government have to stand up and be counted and be held responsible for such criminal acts?

Chapter **35**

DOCTOR'S BLUNDERS

If you look at the year on year **BLUNDER** figures within the NHS there is no evidence that such blunders are teaching doctors or their management very much. We all know that the greater majority of doctors do a first class job and I would be the first to agree with that. But if this book does nothing more than make doctors and those who manage them more accountable to the public then it will have been well worth the countless hours that went into writing it. Throughout this book when I refer to **doctors** I'm really referring to those doctors that know that they are a liability to their patients and to their profession.

I'm referring to the **dead wood** that is found in all such large organisations that lives off the fine work done by their colleagues. These are the doctors that should be weeded out not just for the patient's sake but also for the good name of medicine. It's not enough to expect a doctor to openly report his/her colleague's mistakes to management (The BMA or the GMC) we all know this method is totally inadequate because of misplaced loyalty or fear of reprisal. The British Medical Association are much like a doctor's union, they try to support and inform doctors. But the GMC is supposed to be there to serve and protect the public *(the patient)* from unscrupulous and incompetent doctors. What I would suggest in the first instance is that a *confidential* phone line be set up so that a doctor's incompetence could be easily brought to the attention of these regulatory bodies.

WHY DOCTORS DON'T MAKE YOU HEALTHY.

Source: Daily Mail of Tuesday 9th January 2001

Professor Liam Donaldson the governments Chief Medical Officer specified in his report on N.H.S. blunders that **40,000** deaths per year are attributed to **mistakes** made by doctors. That's an average of **109 people a day** that enter hospital in Great Britain and **die**... as a result of a **BLUNDER** made by one of our highly trained and professional doctors. (In the US they kill off an average of **800 patients** a day...*source: Ralph Nader.*)

We're not talking here of patients that died through trauma from a road accident or such where doctors did their best but could not save them. We're talking here of patients that died due to the fact that the **doctors** were incompetent. Imagine a train or plane crash **every single day** that kills over a hundred people; do you not think that questions would be asked? We all know for sure that there would be a **major** investigation and that heads would roll. So why does this not happen in the world of medicine?

Is this a planned action *(or lack of it)* by the Establishment and the GMC? Is it a huge protection racket? I won't go into detail here for you will read in the following pages of the unworkable procedures that swing into action to protect doctors if anybody should dare to complain.

The N.H.S. has a litigation fund of **taxpayer's** money to the tune of **£400 million** *(each and every year)*. This money is used to pay legal fees and damages when cases are brought against them. Why should taxpayer's money be used to pay damages to patient's families on behalf of the doctors that kill patients due to incompetence? Surely the doctors that committed these crimes should be made to pay from their own pocket and if found guilty of manslaughter which this would presumably be, then as with anyone else a custodial sentence should be considered. At the very least they should be struck off the medical register for gross incompetence and kicked out of the profession for good.

It's not just James Bond that's licensed to kill!

It's a shame that here in the West we don't have a similar medical system to the one in China where doctors only get paid if you're healthy. They are after all the so-called professionals that we pay to **make** and **keep** us healthy so why should they get paid if we are sick? On that same basis if a doctor prescribes a medication and it doesn't work then surely it would not be unreasonable for us to expect a full refund of the prescription cost.

I was born in 1947 and as a child I remember very well how my parents and other working class people of that era respected doctors. As the years rolled by we have all come to realise that these people are not gods, they are human just like you and me. And just like you and me they are out there trying to make a living in order to pay their bills. In the days of the class system up to the end of the Second World War working class people were mostly kept ignorant by those who ruled them. There was no such thing as college or university for the children of workers as those privileges were reserved strictly for the toffs. So people like my mum and dad had to bow and scrape to the more fortunate members of society such as doctors in order to get what they assumed would be a better and healthier life for them and their children.

Oh!…How history has proved that assumption so wrong.
The prescribing of harmful and unnecessary drugs has ruined the health of many generations. Drugs that were prescribed by the very people who were entrusted to look after us.

WHY DOCTORS DON'T MAKE YOU HEALTHY.

Source: Sunday Express 12th December 2004

*Three quarters of a million people are admitted to hospital every year suffering from bad reactions to their medicines - filling the equivalent of **32 entire hospitals**. The problem costs the NHS **(us the taxpayer)** £466 million pounds a year. On any given day 6.5 per cent of the total NHS bed capacity is being used up by patients suffering a bad reaction to medicines prescribed by their GP.* This information came from a study by Liverpool University.

I guess Liverpool University won't be getting anymore drug company research grants. That'll teach 'em not to come up with this stuff in future!

These are huge numbers. I'm not saying here that most doctors are corrupt or go around making wrong decisions that incarcerate or kill people. What I am saying is that doctors should have to answer for their actions in an *(open)* independent inquiry or court of law and if found guilty they should be punished like everyone else.

If those that run the world of medicine from within are not seen to be addressing this problem fairly and in an open and responsible manner with account for the interests of **all** parties involved, then it's hardly surprising that private legal action is taken by relatives of those that the doctors have maimed or killed through gross incompetence.

It's quite clear that governing bodies have blatantly over protected both their own interests and those of the doctors since the NHS was set up. To prove what I have just said take a greatly reduced figure of 50 **avoidable** deaths per day *(that's 50% less than those publicly admitted to by the Chief Medical Officer)* and ask what action if any has been taken against those incompetent doctors that have **killed** up to **1,000,000 (ONE MILLION)** patients over the last 50 years. And do please remember that these figures are based solely on the number of deaths caused by **doctor's blunders** which have been **admitted** by the medical profession. It's a brave man or woman that would hazard a guess as to what the true figure is.

A word of advice to the NHS untouchables in these days of US style lawsuits. It would be an unwise management and/or doctor that ignored this warning. The day is coming when you will have to stand up and be counted just like the rest of us.

The NHS is the biggest employer in the UK with an annual turnover of taxpayer's money of some £94 billion pounds.
Source: The Independent. 18th January 2006.

God knows how much it costs to train a doctor over 7 years.

But who teaches doctors?

Doctors teach doctors. So warts and all are passed on into that knowledge hungry **brain** of the new medical student. Many good practices will of course be learned by the student whilst at medical school but so too will many bad practices, as the student has no choice but to accept what their peers teach them. Once qualified they go off into this big wide world with a prescription pad in one hand and a new stethoscope around their neck, now ready to heal the masses and work till they drop. Of course we need doctors and drugs but if medical students were trained in Electro-Dermal Screening (EDS) which is what I do at Health Scan then we wouldn't need 80% of them because the vast majority of the people would be healthy.

Whichever way you look at it there would be massive savings made and an awful lot of people that are now suffering would be cured. One could also reasonably ask why it is that my work has been almost totally ignored by the doctors of the 10,000 patients that I have treated and cured. Why have only a few doctors ever approached me? If this is not an excellent example of the fact that a great many doctors do not have their patients best interests at heart then what is?

NHS management, doctors and politicians have a lot to answer for.

Source: Daily Mail Friday 2 March 2001
One in every ten NHS patients can expect something to go seriously wrong, and two out of every ten of these patients can expect to be permanently injured.

The Department of Health has confirmed these figures.

If this were a garage would you take your car in for repair?

The cost *each year* to the NHS *(us taxpayers)* of caring for patients that have been injured by the very people that were supposed to cure them is:

£1 BILLION

It is estimated that this money would pay for 3 million days of treatment for people that **should** be in hospital.

What is going on?

2002...Daily Mail headline of Wednesday June 29th

"WE MUST ACCEPT NHS ERRORS" SAYS MINISTER

Well I've got news for you Lord Hunt we **don't** have to accept these countless NHS errors. The public are being **killed** in large numbers **every day** by your incompetent staff and you have the audacity to tell us that we have to accept it! Let me remind you who pays your wages and the wages of all your politician friends.

Oh!...And by the way the medical profession are not learning from mistakes as stated by The Department of Health when NHS blunders killed 34,000 patients in 2001.

In 2002 they killed 40,000 patients!

I'm not saying here that all of these cases were doctor's blunders but you can bet your life that most of them were. So, when patients are admitted to hospital even for minor problems there's a very high risk of them never coming out again. It's a one way trip to the mortuary for **40,000** or more of them.

Some healthcare system that is!

Chapter 36

HARLEY STREET

I've worked at a few different addresses in Harley Street over the years, I understand the image thing and that most doctors one-day dream of being a Harley Street specialist. Harley Street is supposed to be the pinnacle of the medical world and only the so-called best doctors are expected to attain such heights.

Well let me tell you that this is not the case. Of course there are many very good doctors in Harley Street but there are also some very questionable ones too.

Many times whilst working in Harley Street I found it quite difficult to identify just were the doctors and who were the patients. Often I would see an elderly man struggling up a lusciously carpeted staircase arm in arm with another man or woman and the one that looked to be in the worst condition quite often turned out to be the doctor. Very few doctors have full time rooms in Harley Street. Rooms are mostly rented by the hour or by the day, depending upon how many patients you have to see. There are so many doctors coming and going all day that you very rarely get to know anyone. Many times I have seen doctors rushing in the back door of the building as their patient is coming in the front. This happens in reverse also, often the doctor would be out the back door and off in his/her car before their patient had even left the building.

One thing that has always confused me is:
If a doctor can cure you in Harley Street when you're paying incredibly high fees then why can't that same doctor cure you in

your local hospital? As most Harley Street specialists will also be working for the NHS as surgeons etc…(or *is Harley Street just a nice little earner on their day off?)* The more I've treated and spoken with patients that have been to Harley Street for medical help the more I've come to realise that even there a **cure** is more often an illusion than a reality. Most people go to Harley Street as a last resort because the NHS has failed them and as I've just said the crazy thing is that the very doctor that failed them in the NHS could well be treating them in Harley Street. You would be amazed at the amount of doctors I have treated for their own health problems both in Harley Street and elsewhere over the years. Doctors are only human you know and if they can't cure your health problems then how can they cure their own?

I remember my first morning in Harley Street, my illusion of grandeur was well and truly shattered. I was sitting at my desk in my very expensive suit thinking how well I had done to get this far and wishing that my mum and dad were alive to see me, as they would have been so proud. Imagine my disillusionment when I opened two drawers of the desk in the room I had rented for half a day. One drawer was empty apart from a badly rusted stethoscope and the other was half full of mouldy fruit and sandwiches.

Chapter **37**

CONTROLLING THE CONTROLLERS
The General Medical Council
The Medicine Control Agency
and
The Advertising Standards Authority

You would not believe the amount of controllers that exist today in the world of medicine. Fat salaries are paid to the managers of countless hospitals and other organisations that are supposed to be protecting our interests by ensuring that we **the taxpayer** receive a fair and efficient healthcare system. We will also be taking a look at the drug companies as they are a **major** benefactor of NHS funds and as such they have a large input into the day to day running of the organisation.

The sale of drugs from these legal drug barons to the NHS brings in **over 10 billion pounds** each and every year to pharmaceutical coiffeurs (*source: The Independent 18th January 2006*) and with this in mind there are a great many people within such companies that have the sole task of ensuring that NHS doctors and management are kept happy. As the foreword of this book explained doctors are offered many financial inducements for prescribing sufficient quantities of this that or the other medicine. If doctors are offered such things for **their** individual roles then what might be offered to a **bulk buyer** of an NHS trust?

Any such approach by a company to a representative of our healthcare system should be an offence punishable by law *(just as it would be if you tried to bribe a police officer)* and acceptance of any such inducement should also be punishable by law.

If such bodies are permitted to offer inducements to promote their products then how can we the public expect to receive drugs that not only do the best job but are also cost effective.

Doctors, Health Ministers and any other influential public health employees should not be allowed to own pharmaceutical shares and these same people should be banned from becoming employees of drug companies once they leave their current employment. Have any ex-Health Minister's, Hospital Managers or Politicians taken a seat on the board of any drug company in the last 50 years? If so can this not be considered suspicious and possibly detrimental to the interests of the public that previously employed them?

How much public funding *(taxpayer's money)* is given to these legal drug barons for research purposes every year?

How much of this money is invested by drug companies into research at our universities each year?

If drug companies invest large sums of money into research at such establishments then no doubt they monitor and control the published test results. As mentioned earlier in this book drug companies have no legal obligation to reveal results of such testing. Can this be considered safe and in the public interest?

Just stop and read the (*published*) side effects of your medication before taking it, you'll find it on the leaflet that accompanies the drugs. *(also worth a look on the internet).* Most drugs have major side effects that can and do cause numerous other health problems (just look back at Seroxat & Prozac on pages 139 & 140) If you stop to check the known side effects you may well consider it a better option to put up with the health problems you have rather than risk a multitude of new ones.

WHY DOCTORS DON'T MAKE YOU HEALTHY.

The B.B.C. News of May 19th 2003 reported how Jean-Pierre Garnier Chief Executive of Glaxo-SmithKline the UK's largest pharmaceutical company could have netted £22 million pounds for being sacked.

Well, if this is not society gone mad then what is?

This guy was due to receive £22 million pounds for **not** doing his job properly! If he gets that much for being a failure what are we to conclude?

Was this sum a huge payoff to keep him quiet?

Let's now look at some of these organisations in detail and you can make your own assessment.

NHS managers run an organisation that allows its employees to kill **40,000** patients a year through **avoidable** blunders. The attitude of management would seem to be if we can't cover up the blunder then we'll happily pay damages out of our litigation fund of **£400 million** per year of taxpayer's money.

So one way or the other the problem will be solved.

How do you put a price on a life? Do you really think that such **avoidable** killing of patients would be allowed to continue if management themselves were held personally or partly responsible? Why should they not accept a certain amount of legal and moral responsibility for such blunders, after all they happily accept large salaries for employing the people that make them?

WHY DOCTORS DON'T MAKE YOU HEALTHY.

A report prepared for the government and published in *London's Evening Standard of Friday 21st July 2000* stated: NHS Hospitals are being crippled by shambolic management not a shortage of cash.

***

THE GENERAL MEDICAL COUNCIL

This text was taken from the GMC website:

The GMC is best known to the public through handling complaints or other information which casts doubt on a doctor's fitness to practise. We are not a general complaints body and can only act where there is evidence that a doctor may not be fit to practise. Lesser problems can usually be resolved locally, in particular through the NHS procedures. We have agreements with the Commission for Health Improvement, National Clinical Assessment Authority and the National Care Standards Commission to make sure we work together effectively to protect patients.

We can take action:
When a doctor has been convicted of a criminal offence.
When there is an allegation of serious professional misconduct.
When a doctor's professional performance may be seriously deficient.
When a doctor with health problems continues to practise whilst unfit.
If there is evidence that patients may be at risk we can suspend or restrict a doctor's registration as an interim measure.

***

PROTECTING PATIENTS, GUIDING DOCTORS

These are the words that one sees at the top of their website homepage. We shall now look closer at these claims.

Firstly…I see that the GMC is a charity.

Oh!…That's handy!…So they don't have to pay tax like us poor unfortunate individuals and no doubt like most charities they get a **huge** government grant of taxpayers money each year. How can organisations such as this that are almost certainly financed by the government and allowed to make **tax free** income be in a position to protect the rights of the public? It's obvious that if their masters in Whitehall pay the bills then they **also** pull the strings. If the GMC don't do as the government wants then they're all out on their ear and looking for new jobs. Not paying income tax is only one of many perks that charities enjoy. Not having to pay income tax also leaves more money in the kitty for management's **larger than life** salaries.

That's nice!

As the GMC are supposed to be there to protect us the **patient** from the dangers of the medical world then would it not be reasonable to make it compulsory for all GMC management to divulge any outside interests they may hold in drug companies etc?

200,000 doctors are registered with the GMC in the UK.

The GMC are a public body set up to expose and strike off incompetent doctors

WHY DOCTORS DON'T MAKE YOU HEALTHY.

With 40,000 **avoidable** deaths each and every year how can they claim to be an effective and value for money organisation?
In addition the NHS has openly admitted that there are nearly a million reported **blunders** made on an annual basis. *(How many blunders go unreported?)* These mistakes although they do not kill will in many cases maim a patient for life.

The public has a right to know that our lives and those of our children are in the hands of competent doctors and that those doctors are being managed by competent management at the GMC and BMA. If the GMC are responsible for licensing doctors then why are they not **also** responsible for the blunders made **by** those doctors? Maybe that's the very reason that not many doctors are investigated and/or struck off the medical register. In the rare event when a doctor was struck off the medical register in the past were any members of the GMC also sacked?

IF NOT!...WHY NOT?

That would be an interesting little item to research, my bet is that there will have been very few **if any** such sackings. The GMC's website states that they are now bringing in **'National Performance Appraisals'** to monitor (and improve where necessary) every UK doctors performance. Basically **every** doctor will now have his/her performance reviewed and not as in the past when it was just those that couldn't find a way to cover their mistakes that were investigated. The problem with this idea is that responsibility for monitoring and appraising a doctor's performance will now rest solely with hospital management.

NOW!...IF THAT'S NOT A CASE OF THE BLIND LEADING THE BLIND THEN WHAT IS?

If this wonderful idea was designed to instil confidence in the general public then I've got news for you at the GMC.

IT WON'T!

If such an appraisal is considered beneficial at hospital level then why should it not also be introduced at the offices of the GMC?

How **are** GMC management currently assessed?
Is it in direct relation to the performance of the doctors they control or is it related to the number of doctors that are **struck off** the medical register each year? Well on both counts they have failed miserably. I know it's difficult but do try and remember that the GMC was set up to protect **us** the public from incompetent doctors, they are **not** there to protect doctors.

Um!

Here are more questions that beg answers, as I could see no such information on their website.

Who are the faceless people that make up the GMC?
Who appoints them?
Who sets their salaries and annual increases?
What other perks are being provided?

We the public have a right to know who we are paying to **protect** us from dangerous and unscrupulous doctors. I presume that the GMC have to answer to somebody but I could be wrong, if anybody I guess it's the Minister of Health. If I'm right then has the minister ever questioned the GMC as to just why they continue to allow incompetent doctors to kill **40,000** patients a year?

WHY DOCTORS DON'T MAKE YOU HEALTHY.

We will now dissect some pages from the GMC website and try where possible to read between the lines as I'm more interested in what they're **not** telling us than what they are, my comments along the way are in *italic*.

Protecting the public. *(Did that say 'Protecting' the public?)*
We have strong and effective legal powers designed to maintain the standards the public has a right to expect of doctors.
(When will they start using their powers?)
We are not here to protect the medical profession *(Um!)* their interests are protected by others; our job is to protect patients. *(?)*
The public trust doctors to set and monitor their own professional standards. *(Who said that the public 'trust' doctors to monitor themselves?...nobody asked me!)* In return doctors must give their patients high-quality medical care. *(When will this start to happen?)* Where any doctor fails to meet those standards we act to protect patients from harm, if necessary by striking the doctor off the register and removing their right to practise medicine. Our legal authority is the **Medical Act** which gives us powers to protect, promote and maintain the health and safety of the public.

We are also a charity (registration number 1089278) whose purpose is the protection, promotion and maintenance of the health and safety of the community. *(And tax avoidance.)*

The full Council meets three times a year, in February, May and November. Most of our work is done in committees meeting throughout the year.

How are we made up?
Our governing body, the Council, currently has 35 members.

19 are doctors elected by the doctors on the register.
(How can a doctor be 'neutral' when making a judgement on

a fellow doctor?)

14 members of the public nominated by the Privy Council.
(Who are these people in the Privy Council?)
(How did they get there?)
(How much of our money do they receive?)
(Are the 14 members of the public friends or family of Privy Council members? If not then how are they chosen?)

2 doctors appointed by educational bodies - the universities medical royal colleges and faculties. *(research in such places is mostly funded by drug companies)*

The Privy Council nominees are not medically qualified their task is to speak for the public, enabling the GMC to act as a focus for debate between doctors and patients. They play a vital part in all areas of our work. *(Well they give the public the 'impression' that you're interested in their views, so they serve their purpose)*

***

Let us now turn our attention to those in power that have the overall authority to decide which drugs are permitted to be used by doctors. Organisations such as the Medicines Control Agency and many other faceless individuals who I'm sure are earning vast salaries for their trouble. These people and hospital management have a lot to answer for with regard to the use of **dangerous** medication. I would like to know how they can justify their role in the following reports.

Source: Daily Express Thursday March 30th 2000
Over 2 million children aged 2 or under were vaccinated with potentially infected material taken from cattle at the height of the

MAD COW scare. I doubt if those responsible for these mad cow vaccinations would allow their own children to receive one!

But it's okay for our kids!

Question: Why were these people *(and the drug companies involved)* not all prosecuted for intentional criminal poisoning?

Source: Evening Standard 27th February 1997
Hundreds of medicines routinely given to children have never been properly tested or licensed, while some have not even been approved for human consumption.

October 1997
The investigative ITV programme '**THIS WEEK**' announced in a report that Organic Phosphates which cause brain damage have been prescribed for the treatment of NITS in children.

Source: Daily Express 24th February 2003
A commonly used asthma medication that made asthma worse and was linked to fatal asthma attacks has been withdrawn from the market. A leading British expert said, "*It was likely that this drug was not to blame for these excess deaths."* Ah!...oh well that's okay then we won't worry about it if you say it's **likely not to have killed these people**. What the report doesn't tell us is just who this '**leading British expert**' is or what interest/s he/she may have in drug companies.

Source: Daily Express Thursday February 17th 2000
This report highlights the filthy conditions in our NHS hospitals and the incompetence of management to hire and manage competent cleaning staff. Bugs picked up in hospital **kill** 100 people each and every week! This has nothing to do with the incompetence of the doctors; this is a bug that you pick up due to

the unhygienic conditions of the hospital. The one place you would expect to be clean and hygienic is a hospital. There's a 1 in 10 chance of picking up this bug when you're in hospital.

ITV's News at Ten in July 1998 reported that 60,000 people a year...1,000 or more patients a week pick up infection in hospital. Whatever the true number is it's clear that hospital management do not have the situation under control.

***

THE ADVERTISING STANDARDS AUTHORITY

The following text was taken from their website:

The ASA is the independent self-regulatory body for non broadcast advertisements, sales promotions and direct marketing in the UK. We administer the British Code of Advertising, Sales Promotion and Direct Marketing (The CAP Code) to ensure that advertisements are legal, decent, honest and truthful.

The first thing that is highly questionable in the above is that the ASA is a self-regulatory body. This means that they **do not** have to answer to anybody with regard to their policies and their day to day decisions. Is it possible therefore that certain decisions from time to time may well favour their own personal interests?
If for example the policy makers at the ASA had shares in or were otherwise involved with a company would they be inclined to look leniently at its advertising claims or any complaints made against that company? I think human nature tells us that they would. I have looked carefully at ASA management individuals *(it's all on their website)* and many of them are directors or senior management of National or International companies and these companies are all major advertisers.

Many years ago I had a nasty letter from the ASA. They threatened me with legal action if I didn't stop claiming in my advertising that I could **cure** people. The fact that I **did** cure people was of no interest to them. I offered them hundreds of testimonial letters as proof that I was curing people but they refused to accept them. What right do these people at the ASA have to keep such information from the general public?

In every case my clients had been to see doctors looking for a cure and not found it, that's why they came to me. So when a cure does exist what right have these people to keep it from you?

I wonder what the European Court on Human Rights would have to say about this matter. I don't know what the situation was back then but looking at the ASA management line-up today I do not see one person with any medical knowledge. It's probable that the situation was the same years ago when they stopped me from advertising so I fail to see how they could have come to such a decision. The very least they should have done was to investigate my claims and if found to be legitimate then I should have been allowed to continue with my advertising. Maybe someone from the ASA would be good enough to email me and let me know how certain breakfast cereals, margarines and yogurts can be good for your heart. I presume they will have investigated such claims thoroughly. So much for the work of the ASA (Advertising Standard Authority) here in the UK. Believe it or not they are funded by us the taxpayer to look after our interests and to protect us from such dubious advertising.

Chapter **38**

THE GMC PANTOMIME FOR DEALING WITH COMPLAINTS

Introduction   *(From their website)*

The GMC's Fitness to Practise Procedures are linked to licensing doctors and maintaining the medical register. A doctor's registration can be restricted or removed if one of the 'Fitness to Practise' committees decides that this is necessary.
The GMC can take action against doctors if:

    i)   The doctor has been convicted of a criminal offence.
             (Dr Shipman was a convicted drug addict, yet he was still permitted to practice medicine for many years before being arrested for numerous murders.)

    ii)   There is evidence of conduct that appears to be so serious that it is likely to call into question the doctor's fitness to continue in medical practice
             i.e: serious professional misconduct.
             (A *certain Dr Shipman 'murdered' hundreds of patients...maybe thousands. This notorious serial killer went unchecked in his murderous work for a great many years. Did heads roll at the GMC regarding this case ...If not...Why not?)*

    iii)   There is evidence of a repeated departure from good professional practice whether or not it is covered by specific GMC guidance, sufficiently serious to call into question a doctor's registration.

This is termed seriously deficient performance.

(How many patients is a doctor allowed to kill before the GMC consider it 'sufficiently serious' to investigate?)

iv)   There is evidence that a doctor is not fit to practise medicine because of the state of his or her health.

The GMC's powers are aimed at dealing only with the most serious concerns about a doctor which are likely to call into question the doctor's fitness to practise. There are other procedures in place locally for considering other categories of patient concerns.

Okay!...So lets look through the stages of getting a doctor **struck off** *the medical register and remember that we are talking here about investigating a doctor for one or more blunders that he or she* **has admitted** *making. As you read, it will be difficult but do try and remember that the GMC are there to fight* **our** *case against the incompetent doctor that has just killed or maimed our relative, they are* **not supposed** *to be there to protect the doctor. Remember also that whilst this* **hurdle race** *is going on you the relative will almost certainly be greatly traumatised following the* **avoidable** *death or maiming of your loved one.*

Ready!...They're under starters orders and they're off!

The Collection of Information *(Hurdle Number 1)*

The first stage is for one of the GMC's caseworkers *(The caseworker is a doctor, so here's your first hurdle!)* to assess whether concerns should be investigated further. If, after carrying out an initial assessment it is decided that a case does need to be considered further under one of the GMC's procedures, the next step will be to ensure that all the information required to assess the case properly is available. This will often involve some, or all, of the following:

- A written account of the complaint.
- Copies of any relevant medical records or reports.
- If complaints have been made directly to the doctor or to another organisation, copies of any relevant correspondence.
- When did it happen? There is a cut off time limit after which no action can be taken.

Informing the doctor

Before a formal decision on a case can be taken the doctor concerned will be given an opportunity to comment on the allegations. The GMC will need your agreement to do this, but a case cannot normally go forward without telling the doctor.
You will get a chance to respond to the doctor's comments.

Screening

Once all the information needed has been gathered a case will be considered by one or more council members appointed as 'screeners'.
(Your second hurdle!)
Their role is to consider:

- Whether a case raises concerns about a doctor which are so serious that they need to be referred to the next stage of the GMC's fitness to practise procedures.
- Which of the procedures would be the best way of examining the concerns.

A case will always be considered first by a medical member.
(I think you mean a 'doctor'!) (3rd hurdle!)

If the medical member *(doctor)* decides that no action is required the case will not be closed without the agreement of a second, lay member (that is someone who is not medically qualified).
*(Don't you mean someone who does what their told **if** they want to keep their job?)*
If either the medical member *(doctor)* or the lay member *(friend of doctor)* decides that the case does raise serious concerns it will be placed under one (or more) of the following procedures:

- Conduct
- Performance
- Health

All these procedures are explained in the paragraphs below.
If the members both agree that there is no need for any further action against the doctor the GMC will write to you and to the doctor explaining the decision.
It is not normally possible to appeal against this decision.
*(Now there's a surprise!...So you **could fall** at the 3rd hurdle!)*

How long will this take?

It can take some time to obtain all the information usually needed for the screeners to make a decision. The GMC aims to be able to take a screening decision within six months of receiving your complaint but are often able to do so much sooner. *(So to get here could take 6 months but don't get excited you haven't won yet there's loads more hurdles to jump, in fact the race has only just started. The longer they can drag out the case (race) the more you cool down and the less they will have to pay you if they eventually lose. Oh!...and don't forget that the doctor their investigating is probably still out there treating patients.*
*I wonder how many more he or she has killed and/or maimed? They'd better start working a bit faster as there's been another **20,000 blunder** deaths in the NHS and **400,000 other blunders***

since they started on this enquiry 6 months ago.) If there is evidence that the doctor poses an immediate risk to patients *(The doctor has made a **blunder that's killed or maimed somebody!** I'd say that's an **'immediate risk to patients'** wouldn't you?)* the GMC will ensure that the case is dealt with quickly and will ask the Interim Orders Committee

(4th hurdle!...Yet another committee!...okay how much are these guys costing us?) to consider whether the doctor should be suspended or have conditions on his/her registration while enquiries continue. *(That's nice of them!)*

Conduct Procedure

The GMC's Conduct Procedures *(Pardon!... Who?... What?... 'Conduct Procedures'...What's this... Not **another** committee you've sneakily tried to squeeze in here?...5th hurdle)* consider allegations of serious professional misconduct and deal with doctors convicted of criminal offences. *(What like they did with Dr Shipman the **convicted** drug addict and serial killer?)*

Preliminary Procedure Committee (PPC) *(Hurdle number 6)*

The PPC is a panel of medical *(doctors)* and lay members *(friends of doctors)* which meets in private. *(why meet in private?... if you already have some **lay members** in the room then why can't you have other members of the public also?)*

They meet to consider whether a case should be referred to the Professional Conduct Committee (PCC) *(7th hurdle)* for a full formal inquiry in public. If the PPC decides there is no need to refer the case to the PCC they may still provide the doctor with advice about their future conduct.

*(Did I read that right!.. You say the PPC **'MAY'** provide the doctor with advice about their future conduct?...They've just admitted a blunder that killed or maimed someone for god's sake*

*through gross incompetence!...what advice are you going to give them ...like tell them **not** to report the next one?)*
The GMC will write to you immediately after the PPC meeting to inform you of the decision. *(Thanks!)* The rules which govern the GMC's procedures do not allow for an appeal against a PPC decision. *(**Not allow!**...**who wrote these rules?**...Ops! Careful you could fall here!)* If either screener decides that a case raises a possible issue of serious professional misconduct (SPM) the GMC will write formally to the doctor setting out the allegations against him/her. The doctor then has a further chance to comment before the case is considered by the PCC. The GMC will ask the doctor if he agrees to us disclosing these comments to you.

Professional Conduct Committee
(Hurdle number 7...you are doing well!)

The PCC is the final stage of the GMC's conduct procedures. *(Thank god for that!...How many months are we up to now?)*
Their inquiries are conducted in public *(hooray!)* and the doctor has a chance to respond in person to the allegations.
Before the PCC meets to consider a case the GMC's solicitors will prepare the case by arranging for witness statements, expert reports *(doctors reports)* and any other information needed to bring the case against the doctor. If the GMC asks you to appear as a witness you will be given plenty of warning and your expenses will be paid. *(Thanks!...Would that include a few nights at a posh hotel like when you have your committee meetings?)*
You will need to give your evidence under oath, *(Why!...Is this a court of law?)* you may be questioned by the panel hearing the case and by the lawyer defending the doctor. The GMC understands that for many people appearing as a witness can be a difficult experience and will do what they can to reduce the stress of giving evidence in public. *(Thanks!...Very kind of you.)*

What happens at the end of the case?

If a doctor is found guilty of Serious Professional Misconduct the PCC can:

- Erase the doctor from the register; *(The doctor is guilty of killing or maiming a patient through gross incompetence surely this is the **only** option you can choose or are you going to keep them on so that they can try again?)*
- Suspend the doctor's registration; *(What!...Like for 3 months or so until everything quietens down a bit?)*
- Impose conditions on the doctor's registration; *(You mean something like: '**You're not allowed to kill or maim patients.**')*
- Give the doctor a warning. *(Yeah!...Good idea!...A warning, that'll sort 'em out!)*

If the PCC find that the doctor is not guilty of SPM it may decide to take no action against the doctor *(What!...Even though they have admitted killing or maiming a patient through gross incompetence)* or may issue advice *(?)* about future conduct.
*(So after months and months and zillions of committee meetings and a public enquiry and spending vast sums of public money a doctor that has admitted killing or maiming a patient through gross incompetence may **only** be given a warning! Can this be possible? Who makes these one sided rules?)*

Performance Procedure

The GMC's Performance Procedures assess doctors whose performance appears to be seriously deficient. If the GMC receives information that suggests a doctor may be performing poorly *(**Performing poorly?...For the love of god man!...They're killing people!**)* they will first need to establish whether there is a case to answer. *(Here we go again!)* If there is a case the GMC will invite the doctor to undergo an assessment of their skills and knowledge. *(That's nice don't sack the doctor just **invite** them to an assessment of their skills and knowledge! Why do you need to **assess** them they've just admitted killing or maiming a patient through gross incompetence? ...Their seriously lacking in **skills** and **knowledge** and should surely be removed from the register while manslaughter or other charges are considered?)*

If the doctor refuses to participate or undergo an assessment they will be referred to the Assessment Referral Committee (ARC). *(Ah!...another blooming 'costly' committee!...I hope they have plenty of chairs at the GMC, or is this another posh hotel doo?*

The ARC has power to direct the doctor to undergo an assessment within a fixed period of time. Anybody who has reported the doctor to us would have the opportunity to be heard at the ARC meeting. To carry out the assessment the GMC will send a team of trained assessors to study the doctor's performance. The assessment team will normally include two doctors from the relevant speciality and a member of the public.

(You *mean two doctors plus one friend!)*

The assessment will cover the doctor's:

- Attitudes
- Knowledge *(That shouldn't take long!)*
- Clinical and communications skills
  (This will take even less time!)
- Clinical records and audit results

After the assessment the team will report to the case co-ordinator a medical member of the council *(another doctor)* who supervises the performance cases.

The case co-ordinator will decide on the next step.

This may be:

- To take no further action if the assessment has revealed no serious performance problems. *(But there wouldn't have been an assessment in the first place unless there was evidence of serious performance problems!...or am I missing something here?...I'm still talking about the doctors that **kill 40,000** patients a year and maim thousands of others. I see no difference between your **assessment** investigation and that carried out by the PPC.*

*(Or are you saying that your **assessment** committee only looks at the 'minor' stuff of the **800,000** or so annual **blunders** that doesn't **kill or maim** patients but only slightly injures them?)*

- To ask that the doctor take's action to improve his/her performance if the problems have been identified but they pose no risk to patients.
  *(Oh!... So you're going to '**ask**' the doctor... That's nice!)*
- To refer the doctor to the Committee of Professional Performance (CPP)

(Oh god!...Another dam committee!... More expense!... When will it all end?...It's no wonder our taxes are going through the roof!)

If serious problems have been identified the CPP may if necessary suspend or place conditions on the doctor's registration.

(Yeah!... Yeah!... Yeah!...would somebody please just remind me quickly, is the GMC on our side or the doctor's side?)

(Who won the hurdle race?)

(Oh!...I can't keep up with this...I'm going to put the kettle on)

(10 minutes later)

- After two years registration may be suspended indefinitely. (Ah!...nice cup of tea!...now where were we?)

  Complainants are usually unlikely to be required in person at a hearing unless they express a wish to attend.
  *(Well...if the complainants not there then it's easier to come to a favourable decision... if you know what I mean... **Wink! Wink!** Anyway they'll only spoil the meeting by asking awkward questions.)*

Further details of our performance procedures are available on our website.

(Yeah!...Great!...Yawn...Yawn...where's my biscuits?)

Health Procedure

The GMC's Health Procedures can be applied if a doctor is trying to practice despite being seriously affected by ill health. *(There's lots of unhealthy doctors in Harley Street...why don't you look up there for some?)*
The main aim is to protect patients, *(?)* however, the GMC also encourage the sick doctor to seek treatment with a view to returning to work if possible. The most serious cases are reported to the Health Committee, *(Have we had this one before?...I don't think so!...I can't honestly remember!...**God!...I've got committees coming out me ears!**)* which can suspend or place conditions on the doctor's registration. *(Yawn...is there much*

*more of this?...Ah! maybe I'll just drop the case!...Maybe I was wrong!...Maybe the doctor didn't kill my wife after all! It was probably the hospital cleaner!...**Yes!...that's what happened!...it was the cleaner!**...I need more tea!)*

Interim Orders Committee

(Ah!... Come on lads!...A joke's a joke but don't keep on with this committee nonsense!)

(Hold on a minute though...On second thoughts!...Could I get a job on one of these committees and earn loads of money and stay in posh hotels and pay no tax? It sounds like a great life! I could be one of those 'doctor friends' that go around with clever people and do as they are told!)

Chapter **39**

THINGS TO THINK ABOUT

In all my years of scanning for intolerance I have not found 'E' numbers *(Colourings in food)* to be much of a problem, every now and then they cause a few problems but it's very rare and I've tested about 10,000 people. I know that books and so-called health professionals will tell you that 'E' numbers are bad *(Causing hyperactivity in children for example)* but they **also** tell you that fruit and vegetables are good for you.

Stress!
You don't get stressed if you don't poison your brain.
There's something like 40 million working days lost each year in the UK due to stress. When you don't poison your brain it can cope with everything that comes at it, it wakes up and you feel **great** every second of every day. You only get stressed when your brain is taking in or sending out wrong signals because everything then becomes more difficult to cope with.

Decaffeinated coffee!
How much is it decaffeinated... 10%...20%...30%?
I've looked at the labels on major brands and I can't see any reference to caffeine levels. This could well be clever labelling by the manufacturers who make vast fortunes from people being hooked on this stuff. I would presume that most people buy **decaffeinated** to avoid caffeine. So there you are drinking your de'caf and thinking you're in control of the situation, you've now got off that nasty caffeine stuff and you smile as you think *'the coffee people are not selling me anymore drugs.'* But hang on a minute, if there was no caffeine in it as it would seem we are

supposed to believe then surely the label would not say decaffeinated but:

Caffeine Free!

What about 'ORGANIC' and 'NATURAL' foods surely they're okay? Now there's a question I've been asked hundreds of times. Heroin is organic and natural and I doubt that you would want to put **that** into your body. They're just two words that sell a lot of products and allow retailers to charge more. Personally I feel that they should sell these foods cheaper as they don't do anything to them. I test **organic foods**, its pure organic signals that are programmed into my computer and if the organic foods that I test are poisoning your brain then what chance does your brain have once they start spraying them with chemicals?

Nicotine! That must be one of the **biggest** causes of health problems? Yes, I'm sure it is, but you could count on one hand the amount of times I've found it to show as an intolerance in the brain. Mind you as we all know it doesn't do your lungs any favours and you only get two of them.

Cod Liver Oil - Evening Primrose Oil - Green Tea - Herbs
In general I have found that people who use these on a regular basis tend to become intolerant to them. I can never understand why people drink Cod Liver Oil to help their joints. Surely it would get to their joints far quicker if they rubbed it in?

Even if I find people are not intolerant to Cod Liver Oil or other oils I always advise them not to use them on a regular basis. There's more than enough oil in our daily food for the body's requirements. Apart from a high risk of intolerance another reason I advise against oil supplements is that oil coats the lining of the digestive tract and forms a barrier so food cannot pass through into the bloodstream as efficiently. It causes food to go **through** the body rather than **into** the body and therefore much of what your body requires from the food will be passed out in your faeces.

When you don't poison your brain with drugs called food you become healthy! So why do you need remedies such as oils or anything else?

Remember what I said earlier:
You get healthy by **not** putting things into your body!
You get healthy by **identifying** and **removing** the things that are causing the problem!

IT'S AS SIMPLE AS THAT!

And if you don't have a problem then why do you need a
so-called remedy? But if you go to your GP and come out without a prescription then you'd wonder why you went in. Patients *(and doctors)* have been conditioned *(brainwashed)* into looking for a pill or a cream that will solve a problem rather than removing the cause.

I have had the following reply thousands of times when asking a patient why they are taking this that or the other so-called remedy, *"Well because 'They say' it's healthy."* Is the answer I invariably get.

WHO ARE '*THEY*'?

It's not just good marketing really its brainwashing!
If you tell people enough times that something is good for them then sooner or later they will start to believe it.

WHY DOCTORS DON'T MAKE YOU HEALTHY.

The other answer I sometimes get is:
"Well my friend told me she feels great on it."
Yes okay!...It might well suit your friend's brain but will it suit yours?

***

And nothing to do with diet but did you realise:

That the UK Ambulance Service is **not** considered to be an Emergency Service?

Police and Fire are classified as emergency services by the government but the ambulance service is not. The effect of this classification is to undermine the vital and often dangerous work done by our emergency crews and permits employers to pay peanuts to those that do such an important job. I hope that the Prime Minister and/or Health Minister considers re-classification of such a vital service when next they need an ambulance to save the life of their wife or child. Such re-classification would pave the way for the men and women of this highly skilled and professional service to earn a reasonable living wage instead of having to scrimp and scrape year after year (as I did) to pay their bills because of their dedication to the work that they do.

Pensions
You spend all your working life paying into a state pension.
So if you die before pensionable age why should that money *(Your money)* not be returned to your family?

Our Friends the Drug Companies

Source: Skytext Monday 12th September 2005

Up to 12 senior drug company executives are likely to be charged with defrauding the NHS of more than £100 million. According to THE TIMES, the employees from six firms will be accused of price fixing of commonly prescribed drugs. If convicted the companies could be fined millions of pounds and the individuals jailed for up to 10 years. Two of the firms - GENERICS UK and RANBAXY have already compensated the NHS for a total of more than £16million without admitting liability.

On a Channel 4 programme of 29th December 2005 the celebrity Chef Jamie Oliver was reviewing the outcome of his work with a few schools in the London area in his attempt to bring healthier food to the children. He had previously trained several cooks in preparation and presentation and the programme had been running for a few months. Whilst talking with the school staff they reported that since the children were on this programme those that had previously been using daily inhalers for asthma now no longer needed them. There had also been a dramatic improvement in both pupil concentration and mood swings within the classroom. This outcome was a surprise to all and had been achieved by chance with a random change of diet of school meals.

Could you imaging therefore just how beneficial it would be to a child *(or anyone else)* if they were to follow a tailor made diet *(a computerised Health Scan diet)* 24 hours a day.

PART 5

THE MEDIA CONSPIRACY

Chapter **40**

THE MEDIA

The Media has a responsibility to keep the public informed.
They should inform the public of this advanced computerised
technology for the public have a right to know that a simple
drug free cure is available for most of their health problems.

In fact I would go so far as to say that media personnel are both
morally and ethically bound to report such a story to their
readers/audience so that they can make their own assessment just
as doctors should be ethically and morally bound to inform their
patients. The media should be there to serve the public with true
and factual information and not to facilitate drug companies in
their quest for vast profit. For reasons best known to themselves
*(And my guess is it's something to do with drug company
'advertising' budgets)* the media in general have to a great extent
ignored my approaches over the years. We've had a hundred
years or more of being treated with pills and potions and as a
result all we've managed to do is to create some of the most
profitable companies in the world. As I said earlier if you look at
it from a business point of view why would any pharmaceutical
company want to cure you? **They wouldn't! Because they don't
make money out of healthy people!** Paracetamol is a good
example of what I'm saying and how drug companies keep
making money from you. It's a product that just relieves your
headache, so when your headache comes back next week you
have to buy some more. If we are waiting for drug companies to
educate the public with regard to this **drug free** food intolerance
testing then we are going to be waiting a very long time.

In fact you and I know that it will never happen. The Media should be asking many of the questions raised throughout this book, especially those with regard to doctor's blunders and the GMC. The first major network or publication that sets out to fully investigate this subject will have a story that will change the face of medicine forever and audience and reader figures that they could only have previously dreamed of. The media quite rightly are very fast when it comes to reporting on terrorist attacks on our cities, train and aeroplane crashes and such major incidents that kill 30 or 40 people or more. So why do they not focus in the same way on the fact that incompetent NHS doctors are killing more than 100 patients a day in our hospitals? At least 40,000 patients a year die at the hands of these so called professionals yet we see little or no reporting of such cases.

I have had some media coverage over the years. They mostly approached me to do a one off article or TV/radio interview as a result of seeing how I cured one of their staff or friends. I've also done various PR pushes from time to time and I always felt that there should have been a better response considering that my letter was always accompanied by masses of testimonial letters CD's and DVD's about my work. Appendix 3 shows some of the Newspapers and Magazines that have been good enough to feature Health Scan and I thank them for that. However, a **'one-off'** editorial or a local TV/radio interview *(of which I have done many)* although appreciated is of very little use when it comes to getting the message across. What I need is a chance to prove this technology with a regular weekly health programme on an English speaking National/International TV or radio station. I've just recorded a series of 15 half hour health programmes for a major Arab TV station so things are looking good as far as the Middle East is concerned. I know that if I can get my message out to the people this technology will instigate an incredible change of direction in the world of medicine. The sick will no longer be seen by many in the medical world as a means of generating vast wealth and doctors that do not adapt to this drug free treatment will be left out in the cold.

As I'm now heading towards the end of this book and as were talking 'media' I'd just like to say sorry to a certain reporter at The Daily Express. I suppose I have given her a bit of a hard time really, especially as she's written a very nice *(whole page)* article about me. But this case is a good example of how most of the media have handled this vitally important subject over the years. They seem to think that writing a **single** article or doing a **one-off** TV/radio chat is sufficient. Whilst I do of course get lots of people booking scans as a result of having heard of me in this way the average person would probably think that what I'm saying sounds too good to be true and human nature being what it is many will choose not to listen. It's the follow-up interviews that really get the message across, when they see and hear from patients I've cured. What really bugs me though is when the media don't bother to reply to my letters or emails, even though I may have been following up on an article that they published or presented on a radio or TV show

Examples would be producer's etc on chat/health shows such as BBC's The Morning Show...BBC's Breakfast Show...various CNN programmes, Laura Lee the US lady interviewer and Cassie Braben at the BBC. *(Although I did eventually squeeze a reply out of her on my second attempt)* She produced a programme called **'Food Police'** and I emailed her regarding a girl with Crohns Disease who she featured on a programme that had just been screened. I don't know about you but if I was a staff producer at the BBC and received an email like this *(next page)* I'd be straight into my manager's office and demand that I be allowed to follow it up. Cassie did at least reply to me so I suppose that's something, it didn't do the **billions of people** suffering around the world much good though.

Here's an extract from the email I sent to her:

Hello Cassie,

Having watched Food Police last night I felt that I had to contact you. I phoned B.B.C. Information in Belfast and they kindly gave me your email address. Firstly let me say that Charlotte the young lady with Crohns Disease should not be on antibiotics and/or steroids as these will in the long term make her condition worse. You would think that having studied Crohns Disease for some 10 years (**at taxpayer's expense**) Professor Herman Taylor would have been able to offer a more effective and reassuring solution when speaking with Charlotte and her mum. The best that Charlotte can hope for according to Prof. Taylor is two years of antibiotics and steroids and/or a colostomy bag for the rest of her life. Charlotte does **not** have a problem with the MAP bug as Prof. Taylor stated. Charlotte has a simple **YEAST** infection and I am 100% certain that I can cure her completely within a few months without the need for drugs of any kind.

I'm an Alternative Health Practitioner specialising in the field of Food Intolerance. Please do take a look at my website: www.healthscan.co.uk and at the attached press release as this will explain just how my scanning works.

If you would like to advertise on your show for 50 people suffering with a range of general health problems and if you are prepared to film my work then I will scan them all for free and cure them within about two months. Unfortunately drug companies and doctors in general have a vested interest in not advancing this computerised scanning technology as it cures people without drugs, so can I suggest that if we are to proceed then let it be on the basis that we do it on our own. Do not look for guidance from your resident/staff G.P. or medical advisers. This technology can and will become the future of medicine when enough people know of it and what it can do. Between us we can get the message to the world and then the politicians and doctors will have the unenviable task of explaining to the public why they are withholding such technology when it cures so many health problems so simply and without the need for drugs.

Governments are always complaining about the cost of health treatment *(especially the NHS)* this technology would release billions of £'s each and every year that could be put to better use and most of all it will cure generations to come without the need for drugs. This in effect could well be the most important news story of the century and all it would take is about 3 months to put it together. If you want to work with me then I will be happy to send on a vast amount of P.R. material as well as recordings of radio & TV interviews that I have done over the years. To date such interviews have been on small local stations so their impact has been restricted but if we can show the world my work on the B.B.C. then we will change the global healthcare system for ever.

....

After hearing nothing I emailed her again one week later, on the 20th March, 2003.

WHY DOCTORS DON'T MAKE YOU HEALTHY.

Hello Cassie,

Having emailed you on 13th of March I am still waiting to hear from you. Can you at least acknowledge receipt of my email please. Hopefully you as an investigative journalist will choose to look closely at what I have sent you. The public have a right to know of this technology and its ability to cure most everyday health problems without the need for drugs.

If you choose not to proceed will you please be good enough to let me know why.

Regards,

GERARD KIELTY I.R.B; I.D.E.
....

Her reply some 2 weeks later and dated 3rd April 2003 stated:

"Unfortunately I am not able to take your information any further because I am now working on another programme, nothing to do with The Food Police. I am not an investigative journalist just a BBC staff producer who makes programmes of all sorts. At the moment there are no plans to make another series of The Food Police. Your work does sound fascinating and I am sorry I can't work with you on a programme about it. Thank you so much for contacting me and good luck with your future plans."

Cassie Braben.

So why don't media people like Cassie follow up such stories? Could somebody be applying pressure to prevent them doing it?

If the media don't do their bit then how can we ever get the message to the world? The public need to see true honest and open clinical trials being carried out with independent reporting of the results, such trials can **only** be done via the media.

Any trials that involve Doctors, Drug Companies or Government Health Departments or are carried out behind closed doors will almost certainly be doomed to failure. Let's run such trials in the press or on TV and it will be a brave/foolish politician that will stand up in front of their people and refuse to allow them to have this **'drug free'** treatment.

I am happy to work with world leaders that wish to investigate this technology. Two conditions apply however:

The approach must come from the highest source. I will only respond if world leaders or their closest aids approach me and all such work undertaken **must** receive full media coverage from the onset and be seen to be true and fair.

Chapter **41**

SUMMING UP

According to a report on I.T.V. in September 1998 GP's are among the highest suicide rates in the UK. One in fifteen has a drink (or drugs) problem and they are three times more likely to suffer from liver problems than members of the general public. On average doctors die younger than the rest of the population. So maybe it is not surprising that one in four leaves the profession every year and it is said that if this trend continues there will be few GP's left by the year 2010.

I wonder why they are leaving?

In an attempt to fix the problem the government has approved a pay increase of 26% over the next three years. This will bring a GP's salary up from £65,000 to over £80,000 per year and they will no longer be expected to work at nights or weekends. Very expensive agency staff will (*apparently*) provide cover at these times and hand out the tablets. The cost of this so-called Primary Care has been estimated at some £8 billion by the year 2006. Health authorities have finally admitted that they are running short of doctors as many are disillusioned and leaving the profession whilst others are reaching retirement age. So in an attempt to keep the doctors they have and to attract new medical students the government have resorted to the age-old tradition of throwing money at the problem. No doubt our taxes will rise accordingly in due course.

Why should we put up with such a costly and inefficient healthcare system that not only squanders billions of pounds of our money every year but also allows incompetent doctors to kill and maim patients and then closes ranks to protect them?

We all know that the great majority of doctors do their best for their patients but the fact remains that doctors are not being trained to do the job in a way that cures most health problems. Doctors are trained to prescribe medication and to make vast fortunes for drug companies and others than run their profession. Health Scan technology will free up billions of pounds each and every year in the UK alone. This money could be better spent on the specialisation of doctors to work in surgery and other vital fields of medicine. It could be used to treat patients in the UK instead of having to fly them abroad for treatment in order to get waiting lists down. Some of this money could be used to provide emergency helicopters up and down the country instead of us having to rely on the one or two sponsored helicopters in existence today. Some of this money could be used to provide better salaries and equipment within the NHS or it could be used in the same way within our Schools/Fire and Police Service.

We are talking here of **'billions'** of pounds of taxpayers money *(our money)* being saved each and every year.

We're talking of virtually empty hospital corridors.
Waiting lists will be a thing of the past as spare beds will be available when and where they are needed.

Skytext: Thursday 19th January 2006.
The NHS deficit in England is set to hit £1.2 billion and almost 4,000 health service jobs could be lost.

For far too long now the NHS, a fantastic concept has been run as a closed shop by people with no real interest in its patient's. These people make a fortune year after year from the sick and infirm whilst being protected by their 18th century rules and regulations. Change is on the way whether they like it or not and it's books such as this that will bring about that change. The information contained in this book is universal, it affects all colours and creeds and time will not lessen its validity. If you feel strongly enough about the future of your health service and gross wastage of your taxes then contact your Prime Minister and/or President and demand to know why this **'Drug Free'** technology is not being used in your GP clinics and hospitals. Ask why you and millions of others have to continue to suffer and to take unnecessary and costly drugs when there **is** a simple and effective solution.

Thanks for buying this book. I hope you follow my health advice get healthy and enjoy your life. Please let me have a testimonial email once you become healthy as each and every letter is another step nearer the day when we will see this technology accepted. The powers that be can argue about many things that I say and do in my work but they can **'never'** argue with the results.

Regards,

GERARD KIELTY I.R.B: I.D.E.

intolerance@healthscan.co.uk

www.healthscan.co.uk

APPENDICES

APPENDIX 1

GENERAL MEDICAL COUNCIL WEBSITE LINKS

Right!...If you think the GMC were bad then god help you here.

The following are 'links' I found on the GMC website.
These 80 UK organisations are apparently set up to help us poor patients and to stop doctors injuring about 800,000 of us **'unnecessarily'** every year. That's if we're lucky enough not to be one of the 40,000 they kill. At first sight it would seem that these organisations are there to help us. *(I looked at about a dozen of them)* They all have posh names but if you bring up their websites you'll see that half of them are...yes you've guessed it!

'CHARITIES'

The others with one or two exceptions are financed by the government as they are specific government departments. So it's very much a case of everyone having to keep the government happy if they want to keep there jobs. The bottom line is that no matter **who** you complain to about your doctor you've got almost **no chance** of winning. You'll just go around in ever decreasing circles and probably disappear up the backside of some weird committee or other.

And you know the most ironic thing of all?

We pay their wages!

Links

Action for Victims of Medical Accidents
Association of Community Health Councils for England & Wales
College of Health
Health Service Ombudsman
Long Term Medical Conditions Alliance

National Association of Citizens Advice Bureaux
National Patient Safety Agency
NHS complaints guide
Patient Concern
Patients Association
Patients Forum
Prevention of Professional Abuse Network

Doctors

British Association of Medical Managers
British Medical Association
BMJ Careers Fair
DoctorsNet
Gay and Lesbian Association of Doctors and Dentists
Hospital Consultants and Specialists Association
Locum Doctors Association
Medecins Sans Frontiers
Medical and Dental Defence Union of Scotland
Medical Defence Union
Medical Protection Society
Medical Women's Federation
Refugee Health Professionals Contact Network
Royal Society of Medicine

Education

Academy of Medical Royal Colleges
Association for the Study of Medical Education
Council of Heads of Medical Schools
Faculty of Family Planning & Reproductive Healthcare
Faculty of Occupational Medicine
Faculty of Pharmaceutical Medicine

Faculty of Public Health Medicine
Joint Committee on Postgraduate Training for General Practice
Medical and Dental Education Network
National Advice Centre for Postgraduate Medical Education
NHS Education for Scotland
Quality Assurance Agency for Higher Education
Royal College of Anaesthetists
Royal College of General Practitioners
Royal College of Obstetricians and Gynaecologists
Royal College of Ophthalmologists
Royal College of Paediatrics and Child Health
Royal College of Pathologists
Royal College of Physicians & Surgeons of Glasgow
Royal College of Physicians of Edinburgh
Royal College of Physicians of London
Royal College of Psychiatrists
Royal College of Radiologists
Royal College of Surgeons of Edinburgh
Royal College of Surgeons of England
Specialist Training Authority

General Healthcare

British Medical Journal
British National Formulary
British Psychological Society
Clinical governance support team
Clinical Standards Board for Scotland
Commission for Health Improvement
Complementary Medical Association
Department of Health
General Chiropractic Council
General Dental Council

General Optical Council
General Osteopathic Council
Health Professions Council
Health Service Journal
Institute of Complementary Medicine
Kings Fund
The Lancet
Medical Research Council
Medicines Control Agency
National Clinical Assessment Authority
National Electronic Library for Health
NHS Confederation
NHS Direct
NHS Litigation Authority
National Institute for Clinical Excellence
Nursing and Midwifery Council
Organising Medical Networked Information
Royal Pharmaceutical Society of Great Britain

APPENDIX 2

LETTERS TO WORLD LEADERS AND THEIR RESPONSE

WHY DOCTORS DON'T MAKE YOU HEALTHY.

All world Leaders would do well to take note of this technology. For the gift of **'good health'** is the most precious gift of all and any politician that gives such a gift to their people will be in power for a very long time. The following pages are extracts from letters and emails I sent to Tony Blair, George Bush and John Kerry. There self-explanatory so I will leave you to draw your own conclusions. It is now 2006 and to date the only replies I have had are those you see, I've had nothing from George Bush. I can only assume that these politicians would rather that you their electorate be kept in the dark about this technology. They seem happy to let you suffer with countless health problems whilst they fill their coffers with taxes from drugs and whilst they continue to make drug companies even richer.

You have the power (I assume) Mr Prime Minister and Mr President to change the antiquated, bungling, ineffective and costly world of profit and deceit that is **'Conventional Medicine'** and to open a new era in the world of healthcare.

Here's your chance to serve the people that you represent like no other leader before. Here's your chance to make history and to make a better world for all.

WHY DOCTORS DON'T MAKE YOU HEALTHY.

Sunday 14th December 2003

Dear Mr. Blair,

One single food intolerance test is all that is required to cure most everyday health problems. Drugs are not required in order to bring about a recovery, to do this it's simply a case of finding the cause and removing it. I cure over 50 different health problems this way and have successfully treated about 10,000 people over the last ten years. The enclosed CD/audio and videotapes will fully explain how this technology works.

I will not try to convince you here of the effectiveness of my work for the enclosed material will do that. But just think for a moment; just think how this technology could benefit the British people. If you do introduce it into the NHS it will cure countless millions of patients and save your government billions of pounds each and every year, money that could be better spent on schools and the police, etc.

I will leave it to you to contact me when you are ready.

Please contact me personally as I am not interested in talking with Health Ministers or doctors for many of them have their own selfish reasons to ensure the failure of this technology.

My patients throughout the world include Royal Families as well as household names of sport/stage/screen and politics. If I have not heard from you personally upon my return from Jordan in early February then I shall assume that you are not interested in my proposals.

It's time the British public were informed that there is a simple drug free way to good health and I intend to make sure that they are, hopefully you will be able to work with me on this.

Best Regards,

GERARD KIELTY I.R.B; I.D.E.

10 DOWNING STREET
LONDON SW1A 2AA

From the Direct Communications Unit

19th December 2003

Dear Mr Kielty,

The Prime Minister has asked me to thank you for your recent letter and the enclosures.

Mr Blair receives so many requests of this nature that he has, reluctantly, decided to lend his support in cases only where he has some close personal connection.

Mr Blair has asked me to send you his good wishes for the success of your project.

Yours sincerely

JOHN O'CONNELL

> Reply from the Prime Minister

EMAIL TO PRESIDENT BUSH. *(paraphrased)*

To **BushCheney04@GeorgeWBush.com**
Sent: 04 September 2004 19:54
Subject: HEALTH SCAN
($320 billion healthcare savings in 10 years)

Dear Mr. Bush,
I know that you are a very busy man and that you probably won't get a chance to read my email for a while but I would like one of your staff to reply (rather than me receiving the standard computerised acknowledgement) and let me know that my proposals will be brought to your attention at the earliest possible moment. My work in this field of healthcare is far too important to allow it to be mishandled or downgraded by others that may for one reason or another not wish to see it succeed. So please contact me if and when you wish to move on this. I have proved 10,000 times that drugs are not required in order to cure over 50 different health problems (see list below) all that is actually required to bring about a cure is to find and remove the cause of a problem. Technology now exists to do this work and a single one hour scan is all that's required to cure most people.

You announced on November 3rd 2003 a $4,400 Billion fund to cover US healthcare over the next ten years. Well, I can show you how to save 80% of that money while curing 80% of the people at the same time. I look forward to hearing from you and to working with you in order to bring about these much needed changes and to show the people of America that there is a simple drug free way to good health.

Regards,

GERARD KIELTY I.R.B; I.D.E.

WHY DOCTORS DON'T MAKE YOU HEALTHY.

EMAIL TO JOHN KERRY *(paraphrased)*

To: **info@johnkerry.com**
Sent: 28 January 2004 06:13
Subject: HEALTH SCAN

Dear Mr Kerry,

I have just watched your wonderful acceptance speech.
Listening to you I feel sure you are a man that could go all the way to the White House. I particularly liked your comments on healthcare and your plan to control the drug companies.

I will keep this email short, I can give you the most important tool in your presidential campaign. I can show you how to cure 80% of everyday health problems without the need for drugs of any kind. This would reduce future US healthcare costs by 80% each and every year.

Millions of patients currently suffering throughout America would be cured within a month or so of receiving treatment. I have cured about 10,000 people this way over the last 10 years and can show evidence of curing over 50 different health problems.

Regards,

GERARD KIELTY I.R.B; I.D.E.

WHY DOCTORS DON'T MAKE YOU HEALTHY.

JOHN KERRY'S EMAIL *(REPLY)*

From "John Kerry for President" <info@johnkerry.com
Sent 20 February 2004   22:04
Subject: Reply from John Kerry for President.

Dear Gerard,

Thank you for sending John Kerry your suggestions for the campaign, particularly your insightful healthcare proposal.
With our recent victories and your continued support we are gaining more momentum every day. Your Campaign ideas for John Kerry are very helpful and we will communicate them to the campaign management.

APPENDIX 3

PUBLICATIONS THAT FEATURED HEALTH SCAN

WHY DOCTORS DON'T MAKE YOU HEALTHY.

Here are some of the larger publications that have researched and publicised my work over the last 10 years

SUNDAY TIMES   DAILY EXPRESS

HEALTHY EATING

GOOD LIFE   MARIE CLAIRE

PARENT GUIDE

HEALTH ADVISOR   CAREFREE

AGE CONCERN

SUR (SPAIN)   AL YAQZA

ABSOLUTE MARBELLA

LA VOCE DEGLI ITALIANI   SAYIDATY

GULF NEWS

APPENDIX 4

ABBREVIATIONS USED

BMA	British Medical Association
FDA	Food and Drugs Administration (US)
GMC	General Medical Council
IBS	Irritable Bowel Syndrome
IDE	Investigational Device Exemption
IRB	Institutional Review Board
ME	Myalgic Encephalomyelitis (Chronic Fatigue Syndrome)
MS	Multiple Scierosis
SAD	Seasonal Affective Disorder
SH	Sulphyryl
SNP	Single nucleotide polymorphism
WHO	World Health Organisation

APPENDIX 5

THE TOP 50 PHARMACEUTICAL COMPANIES (2002)

Rank	Company	Headquarters	Sales (billions)	Growth	Share
1	Pfizer	U.S. (New York)	$28.3	+12%	7.1%
2	GlaxoSmithKline	U.K. (London)	$28.2	+8%	7.0%
3	Merck	U.S. (New Jersey)	$21.6	+1%	5.4%
4	AstraZeneca	U.K. (London)	$17.8	+9%	4.4%
5	Aventis	France (Strasbourg)	$17.3	+11%	4.3%
6	Johnson & Johnson	U.S. (New Jersey)	$17.2	+16%	4.3%
7	Novartis	Switzerland (Brazil)	$15.4	+4%	3.8%
8	Bristol-Myers Squibb	U.S. (New York)	$14.7	-2%	3.7%
9	Pharmacia (Pfizer)	U.S. (New Jersey)	12.0	+1%	3.0%
10	Wyeth	U.S. (New Jersey)	$11.7	+7%	2.9%
11	Eli Lilly	U.S. (Indiana)	$11.1	-4%	2.8%
12	Roche	Switzerland (Brazil)	$10.8	+3%	2.7%
13	Abbott Laboratories	U.S. (Illinois)	$9.3	+13%	2.3%
14	Schering-Plough	U.S. (New Jersey)	$8.7	+4%	2.2%
15	Sanofi-Synthelabo	France (Paris)	$8.0	+15%	2.0%
16	Boehringer heim	Germany (Ingelheim)	$7.9	+13%	2.0%
17	Takeda	Japan (Osaka)	$7.2	+4%	1.8%
18	Schering	Germany (Berlin)	$5.4	+10%	1.3%
19	Bayer	Germany (Leverkusen)	$5.1	-16%	1.3%
20	Amgen	U.S. (California)	$5.0	+40%	1.3%
21	Sankyo	Japan (Tokyo)	$3.6	+2%	0.9%
22	Akzo Nobel	Netherlands (Arnhem)	$3.4	+3%	0.8%
23	Eisai	Japan (Tokyo)	$3.4	+21%	0.8%
24	Yamanouchi	Japan (Tokyo)	$3.2	+5%	0.8%

25	Merck KGaA	Germany (Darmstadt)	$3.2	-2%	0.8%
26	Novo Nordisk	Denmark (Bagsvaerd)	$3.2	N/A	0.8%
27	Baxter International	U.S. (Illinois)	$3.1	+11%	0.8%
28	Shionogi	Japan (Osaka)	$3.1	+4%	0.8%
29	Daiichi	Japan (Tokyo)	$2.7	+4%	0.7%
30	Teva	Israel (Petach Tikva)	$2.5	+17%	0.6%
31	Fujisawa	Japan (Osaka)	$2.5	+19%	0.6%
32	Genentech*	U.S. (California)	$2.2	+24%	0.5%
33	Solvay	Belgium (Brussels)	$2.0	+5%	0.5%
34	Purdue Pharma	U.S. (Connecticut)	$1.9	+5%	0.5%
35	Altana	Germany (Bad Homburg)	$1.7	+22%	0.4%
36	Otsuka	Japan (Osaka)	$1.7	+14%	0.4%
37	Tanabe Seiyaku	Japan (Osaka)	$1.6	0%	0.4%
38	Forest Labs	U.S. (New York)	$1.6	+33%	0.4%
39	Serono	Switzerland (Geneva)	$1.5	+12%	0.4%
40	Allergan	U.S. (California)	$1.4	+21%	0.3%
41	Watson	U.S. (California)	$1.2	+6%	0.3%
42	Kyowa Hakko	Japan (Tokyo)	1.2	N/A	0.3%
43	King	U.S. (Tennessee)	$1.2	+35%	0.3
44	Biogen	U.S. (Massachusetts)	$1.1	+10%	0.3%
45	Ono	Japan (Osaka)	$1.1	+5%	0.3%
46	Elan	Ireland (Dublin)	$1.1	-22%	0.3%
47	Alcon Labs	Switzerland (Nueneberg)	$1.1	17%	0.3%
48	Schwarz Pharma	German (Monheim)	$1.0	+25%	0.2%
49	3M	U.S. (Minnesota)	$1.0	+13%	0.2%
50	Genzyme	U.S. (Massachusetts)	$0.9	+9%	0.2%

WHY DOCTORS DON'T MAKE YOU HEALTHY.

Rank	Company	R&D Spend (in billions)
1	Pfizer	$5.2
2	GlaxoSmithKline	$4.3
3	Aventis	$3.7
4	AstraZeneca	$3.1
5	Merck	$2.7
6	Johnson & Johnson	$2.7
7	Novartis	$2.6
8	Roche (not including Genentech)	$2.4
9	Pharmacia	$2.3
10	Bristol-Myers Squibb	$2.2

INDEX

Printed in the United Kingdom
by Lightning Source UK Ltd.
124839UK00001BB/1/A